PRAISE FOR *TUXEN*METHOD

I WAS SUFFERING from what seemed to be more and more of a chronic hip pain. The pain started after a marathon I ran and gradually began to affect my everyday life. Soon I was no longer able to run and had pain in everyday activity such as walking and even playing with the kids. I tried to rest and do exercises, and I tried dry needling with limited effect. The first time I tried the Tuxen Method I felt a burning sensation in my hip immediately after the initial treatment, and the day following I

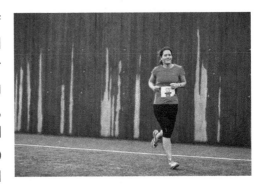

noticed a *huge* difference. In fact, after just after five sessions my hip was *pain free* and I am now active again running marathons and enjoying my life. This is by far the most effective treatment method I have received in my running career. —ELISE, runner, 36

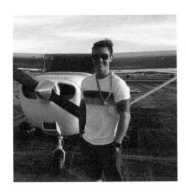

I WAS EXPERIENCEING a backache that started when I was biking for several hours. I also experienced my back pain in my work as a mechanic. I had tried chiropractic, exercise, and had officially given up my cycling career after suffering from back pain for two years before I tried the Tuxen Method. After only two treatments I had greater mobility in my back than I had had in two years. I could feel for the first time in a long time that my back muscles were relaxed when walking and cycling. I am now back on my bike again and working, pain-free, at my job. —MORTEN, cyclist, 26

I WAS STRUGGLING WITH a chronic dizziness and neck pain after being an educator in a kindergarten, working full-time and being a single mother. I was lacking sleep, and in the end dizziness put me on my sick leave. I was not able to take care of my daughter nor was I functioning in my job or everyday life. The doctors said that there was *nothing* I could do, but give it time and give it some rest. After receiving the Tuxen Method to my head and neck it felt like a huge, heavy helmet was removed from my head. I felt more focused and could really feel the blood flow improving in

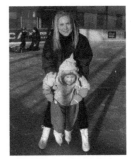

my neck, which previously (and constantly) felt cold and stiff. The Tuxen Method was life saving for me! I am now back at work and feel that I have gotten a second chance to take care of my health. —BRIT JORUNN, child welfare leader, 33

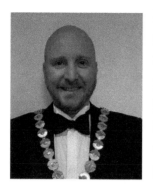

HAVING A LONG CAREER working as a full-time chef, all parts of my body were suffering. I was used to having pain on a daily basis and pain was just a part of my everyday life that I had learned to accept—shoulder pain, back pain, elbow pain, tired legs—these were just a few of my complaints. I was told that this was a price I had to pay to be a chef with a heavy body build. After receiving the Tuxen Method on my whole body I can say with certainty that chronic pain can be removed, even if you have had the pain for several years. In fact I have never felt as healthy nor younger than I do today. —**ATLE**, chef, 39

I HAD SUFFERED from chronic sinus problems ever since my early teenage years and had tried anything I could, from change of diet, conventional medicine, and more, to see if my sinus problems would improve. It was only when I tried the Tuxen Method that I felt a sudden, new, drainage from my sinus. I no longer wake up every morning with chronic sinus pain and dry eyes. When having complaints so long, you don't know how good the quality of your life can be when you don't have your everyday pain anymore. The Tuxen Method has been the *only* really effective treatment I have tried that made an immediate difference to my problem. — **MARIT**, offshore oil worker, 33

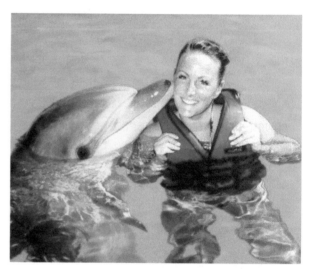

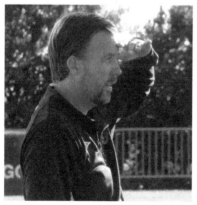

FOR 20 YEARS I played as a professional goal keeper in Scandinavian and Spanish football clubs and I am a professional coach now. Over the years I have suffered from several sports injuries and a lumbar disc prolapse, and of all the treatments I have received nothing compares to the Tuxen Method, in fact I could not have continued in football without the help of the Tuxen Method over these last 10 years. Now that I work as a professional football coach, I always recommend my players use the Tuxen Method as part of the medical support team. Michael Phelps knows what he is doing! —**BO**, 40

TUXENMETHOD

If one way be better than another,

that you may be sure is nature's way.

—ARISTOTLE

TUXENMETHOD

VACUUM & DECOMPRESSION THERAPY

Easy and Effective Soft Tissue Treatment Techniques for Professional Massage Therapists

1st Edition

By

TONJE **TUXEN**

and

SILJE **TUXEN**

Helheten

DISCLAIMER
Care has been taken to confirm the accuracy of the information presented and to describe generally accepted practices. However, the authors, editors, and publisher are not responsible for errors or omissions or for any consequences from application of information in this book, and make no warranty, expressed or implied, with respect to the currency, completeness, or accuracy of the contents of the publication. Application of this information in a particular situation remains the professional responsibility of the practitioner; the clinical treatments described and recommended may not be considered absolute and universal recommendations.

ACKNOWLEDGEMENTS

Thanks to Harald Bjørge for your critical point of view and many questions, and for lifting our book to a whole new educational, clinical reasoning, and scientific level. Thank you for all the countless hours you spent looking at our material. This book would never have been the same without you.

BRIEF CONTENTS

INTRODUCTION

THE TUXEN METHOD DIFFERENCE

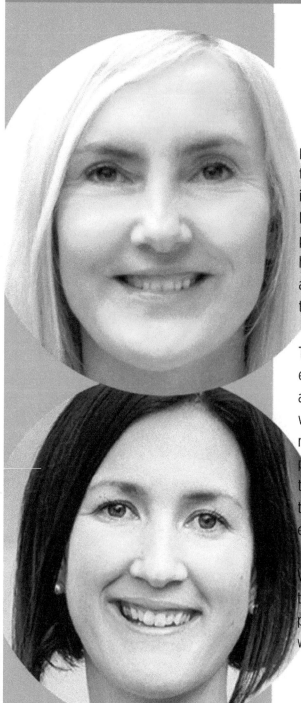

Most of the massage therapy techniques being taught today focus exclusively on the patient, providing approaches to treatment for specific ailments, injuries, and physical challenges. Many of those treatment plans provide valuable methods for healing, but they don't pay any attention to the needs of the therapist.

They leave therapists feeling exhausted and sore day after day, and many therapists question whether their work is really making a difference for their patients at all. As a result, many therapists change careers after they realize how physically and emotionally taxing the job can be.

We recognize the value of your talents, and the value that you provide for your patients. We want to make it easier for you to continue providing the services that your patients need, without having to go home exhausted every night.

We've designed the Tuxen Method with YOU in mind, not just your patients. We want to help you free yourself from the exhaustion and pain that you thought was unavoidable in your career, all while providing top-notch healing opportunities for your patients.

That's why we teach powerful vacuum therapy techniques that allow you to:

- Treat more areas of a patient's body in one session, so that you can provide more help to your patients without exerting more energy;

- Provide dynamic whole-body healing techniques that are perfectly tailored to a variety of ailments and a variety of patients;

- Open up your treatment options into new areas such as anti-aging treatment and metabolic health;

- See more patients every week without exerting more energy as you let the vacuum therapy do the hard work for you;

- And much more!

TONJE TUXEN

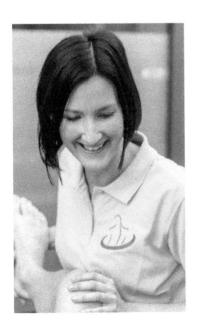

Tonje Tuxen has a bachelor's degree in physical therapy from The European School of Physical Therapy in Amsterdam, the Netherlands. She also has a master's degree in Musculoskeletal Physical Therapy from the University of Melbourne, Australia. Furthermore, she studied one year of health science in Marbella, Spain.

She has long clinical experience working in different clinical settings within the field of musculoskeletal disorders. Tonje has also worked with athletes, both in rehabilitation, injury prevention, and optimizing performance.

Today Tonje runs her own multidisciplinary clinic with professionals from various arts, including physical therapy, manual therapy, chiropractic, acupuncture, osteopathy, running coaching, and nutrition in Stavanger, Norway.

Apart from clinical work, she has worked as a sports instructor and lecturer on injury prevention and healthy living. Tonje is passionate about improving the quality of life for her patients, and employs a holistic perspective to optimize patient outcome.

Tonje has always known she was destined for a career in health, growing up with a seriously ill mother suffering from multiple sclerosis.

Today Tonje shares effective soft-tissue techniques which she developed with her sister, Silje Tuxen.

SILJE TUXEN

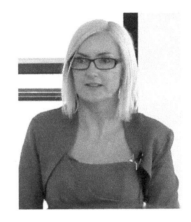

Silje Tuxen has worked full-time as a holistic healthcare practitioner since the late 1990s, and has worked with thousands of children, men, and women of all ages, who have wanted to heal the body naturally.

Before Silje started working in natural medicine she worked for ten years in a large, international oil company, and even though Silje loved that job, her real interest (since childhood) had always been alternative medicine.

Silje's passion for holistic medicine intensified after her mother was diagnosed with multiple sclerosis and conventional medicine could no longer help her, and Silje decided to change professions.

Silje specializes in several alternative medicine methodologies, including nutrition and herbs, reflexology, Thought Field Therapy and EFT, deep-tissue massage, and kinesiology. But the favorite method is vacuum therapy.

We hope to demonstrate why we love this therapy so much, and to effectively teach you the techniques in this book. You can reach us via the contact information in this book. An online certification program in our method is now available as well, which we hope you will avail yourself of. We are excited for you to begin successfully applying the techniques we have found so helpful—even life changing—with our own patients, and to meet you and hear of your own success with Tuxen Method.

Enjoy!
Tonje Tuxen & Silje Tuxen
Stavanger 2016

WHAT IS TUXEN METHOD?

The Tuxen Method is a new philosophy along with a new application of the ancient technique of therapeutic cupping, based on modern physical therapy, massage therapy, and osteopathy. The Tuxen Method is based on a thorough clinical reasoning, integrating knowledge of anatomy, physiology and pathology.

There are several potential benefits of using the Tuxen Method in your clinical practice. These are:

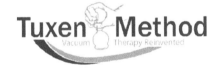

- You will get better results.

- Instead of using your hands, you mostly use a vacuum cup, and thereby decrease the demands on your own body, creating a more sustainable practice.

- You will be able to treat more areas of your client's body within one session.

- You will save time—*lots* of time!

- You will be able to help *more* clients.

- You will increase your confidence as you learn an entire treatment system, applicable on numerous conditions.

- You will gain knowledge of how the different tissues work together and how it all connects, enabling you to prescribe an optimal treatment plan for your clients.

With The Tuxen Method you can treat the same conditions as with conventional massage, but you will be able to expand your area of clinical application and get potentially far better results. The Tuxen Method is also a great tool to combine with traditional massage, as well as with other mobilization and stretching techniques.

OLDER AND OTHER METHODS

Traditional use of *cupping* has been used for a long time (often by unqualified personnel). Traditional cupping is based upon the same philosophy and principles as acupuncture (as with placing cups on acupuncture points) and has been associated with alternative medicine. Either the cups have been used for dry suction only—with a static application, or they have been used as wet cupping—which is a combination of acupuncture and static cupping.

Image: Demonstration of dynamic application of the cup around the back to release the fascia surrounding a muscle. The vacuum cup is connected to a vacuum machine. The pressure can be regulated for the desired effect of treatment.

But with the new Tuxen Method we base our philosophy on science and clinical reasoning, and give a detailed explain what happens on the tissue level. We advocate a dynamic application of the vacuum cups to give a deep-tissue massage effect, and thereby release tension in the fascia; or we use the cups in a static position to release trigger points.

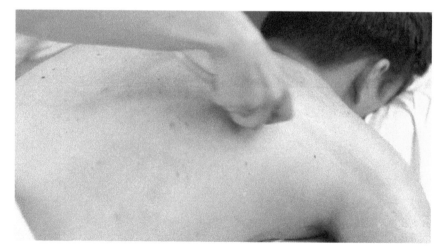

GENERAL RESEARCH ON CUPPING

Since 2010, three studies have investigated the results of cupping on neck pain (Lauche et al., 2011, Cramer et al., 2011, Kim et al., 2012). Lauche investigated the effect of cupping treatments and the resultant effects on pain and mechanical threshold on patients with chronic neck pain. They recruited 50 patients and randomized them into a treatment group plus a wait-and-see/control group. The treatment consisted of five cupping treatments over two weeks. The treatment groups showed significantly less pain and better results on the Short Form Health Survey (SF-36) subscales for bodily pain compared to the control group.

Another study examined the effects of pulsating cupping, and compared this with a control group that received standard medical care. Cramer et al. (2011) recruited 50 patients with chronic nonspecific neck pain and randomized them into treatment plus control groups. The intervention groups were then split into treatment and control groups. The treatment group received five pneumatic pulsation treatments with a mechanical device over two weeks. They found that the intervention group had significantly decreased pain, functional disability (neck disability index - NDI), and quality of life (SF-36). No differences were found in pain at motion and pressure-pain threshold.

Kim et al. (2012) performed a randomized controlled pilot trial to evaluate the effectiveness of cupping therapy for neck pain in video display terminal workers. Forty workers with moderate to severe neck pain were randomly allocated into one of two interventions: six sessions of wet and dry cupping or heat pad application. Both groups received treatments three times a week over a two-week period. The symptoms related to work were evaluated at several points during a seven-week period. The participants were offered an exercise program during the participation period as well. Cupping was found more effective than a heating pad in improving pain (numeric pain rating scale-NPRS), NDI and discomfort (measure yourself medical outcome profile 2-MYMOP score) at two evaluation points (three and seven weeks). Significant improvement in the EuroQoL health index (EQ-5D) was observed at seven weeks in both groups. The researchers found that two weeks of cupping therapy and an exercise program may be effective in reducing pain and improving neck function.

Markowski et al. (2014) evaluated the effects of cupping on pain, tenderness to palpation, and range of motion of patients with sub-acute or chronic lower back pain. Twenty-one patients who had reported back pain for at least eight weeks volunteered to participate in the study. Four glass cups were applied and pressurized over the lower erector spinae muscles. A significant improvement in post-treatment pain scores was found (evaluated by visual analog scale) in the straight leg raising test, lumbar flexion range of motion, and pain-pressure threshold at all four investigated points.

There has been no research of the treatment techniques used by the Tuxen Method. The use of a vacuum-machine instead of manually applying vacuum on the cup itself is a new technique. Research will consequently take several years to be conducted. However, The Tuxen Method is based on the philosophy and science of other soft-tissue techniques within physical therapy and massage therapy.

Hence, some of the ideas and interpretations of the research, are our own. We are fully aware that we don't know exactly what happens when vacuum cupping is applied and why it has such clinical results. We try to communicate to you our ideas and thoughts, but as we all know, research may at a later stage conclude differently. However, the effects of the treatment will be similar, whatever explanation resonates with the updated science.

EFFECTS OF CUPPING

Undoubtedly, the vacuum generated by the cup predominantly affects the epidermis, dermis, and hypodermis. The degree of vacuum that affects the underlying muscle, especially in areas where the dermal layers are thick, is likely small. When applying vacuum therapy on, for example, the lower back, the effect on the erector spina muscle is in all probability quite miniscule. In contrast, when directed at the tibialis anterior, one can more often than not affect the muscle to a larger extent.

But it probably does not matter. As we influence the skin, the ascending pathways of signaling are activated and the brain in all its complexity has descending pathways that in turn can inhibit muscle activation. In other words, a neurological loop exists whereby one can affect muscle tone by stimulating joints, skin, and fascia. This is a more accurate explanation of the effect of the Tuxen Method in large areas of the body.

THE BASICS

[1] CIRCULATORY AND LYMPHATIC SYSTEMS

In order to understand the theoretical background for the Tuxen Method, it is important to have some knowledge of the circulatory and lymphatic systems.

THE CIRCULATORY SYSTEM

The circulatory system consists mainly of the arteries, veins, and capillaries. Blood serves a variety of tasks, including:

- Supply of oxygen and nutrients (glucose, fatty acids, and amino acids);

- Removal of metabolic waste (referred to as waste products in this text) such as carbon dioxide, lactic acid, and urea;

- Transports immunological agents;

- Has a thermoregulatory effect;

- Messages tissue damage;

- Hormone regulation;

- Contributes to pH-regulation;

- And has hydraulic capabilities.

There are certain causes and/or indications of reduced blood circulation and these include:

- Inactivity;

- Smoking;

- Decreased lung capacity;

- Heart/lung disease (these organs are our main "machines" for getting oxygen into our bodies);

- Bluish color in the skin (often seen in the extremities and sometimes in the face and/or lips);

- Cold hands, feet, and other areas of the body can be signs of poor circulation;

- Low threshold of fatigue and/or lactic acid buildup in the legs and/or arms;

- Swollen legs and hands (the lymph system is dependent of the capillaries to work properly);

- Pain or stiffness within several parts of the body can also indicate poor circulation.

A NOTE ON SMOKING

Not many people are aware that smoking not only damages the lungs and heart, but damages the muscles as well. This is because the capillaries deliver blood to the muscles and when you smoke these capillaries tense up and get rigid. Over time you have fewer functioning capillaries and the muscles receive less nutrition and oxygen and cannot remove the waste as well. Additionally, the waste that results from smoking gets captured in the muscles. There is a significant connection between muscle pain and joint pain and smoking. Smoking is much more dangerous than people realize, not only to the lungs and heart but also to the digestive system. There is also a much higher risk of developing rheumatoid arthritis when you smoke—higher even than any genetic risk factor. Also, poor lung capacity increases the risk of tendinopathy.

Reduced blood circulation can be localized within a few muscles (for example, the neck alone) due to high tension in those muscles, or reduced circulation may affect larger parts of the body, such as the upper extremity, lower extremity, or the entire body. It is more typical to have reduced circulation in the parts of the body that are furthest from the heart (such as feet, legs, arms,

hands) and superficially in the muscles, which contain the smallest of the capillaries.

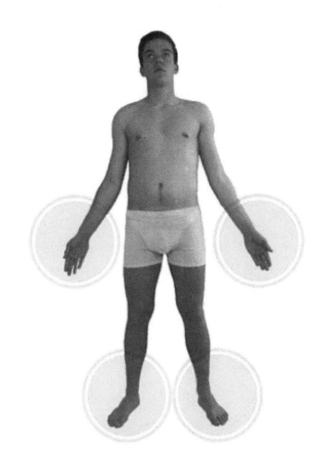

Image 1-1: Cold hands and feet due to poor circulation

WHAT INCREASES CIRCULATION?

The most effective way to stimulate circulation is by exercise, nutrition, and with heat. A combination of these, together with the Tuxen Method, is one of the most effective methods of increasing circulation.

The best exercises are *cardiovascular* exercises, especially high-intensity exercise such as interval training. This improves the performance of the heart (a muscle, after all, which then delivers blood more effectively to the body with each beat). The increased blood flow has a positive effect on the function of existing capillaries and it may also increase the *number* of capillaries by inducing the formation of *new ones*.

People who exercise (especially if *intensively*) normally enjoy better circulation than those who do not exercise, but professional athletes who exercise *constantly* might *develop musculo- skeletal problems* because of repetitive and high load over time. This can in turn inhibit blood flow and hamper performance.

The Tuxen Method is an effective way to help a patient improve his or her blood, apart from exercise and nutrition.

We can and we have compared treatment modalities that increase circulation with the use of infra red cameras (used prolifically in our practice) and nothing improves one's infrared imaging more (or more permanently) than vacuum therapy, especially when it is done using the principles of The Tuxen Method you are about to learn.

In summary, *tense* muscle might lead to a reduced flow of blood in the capillaries and inhibit capillary function. Fewer functioning capillaries will lead to diminished nutrition and scarcity of oxygen to the muscle, which in turn increases pain in the muscle and leads to increased chances of tendon and joint problems. The Tuxen Method *breaks down* old capillaries and stimulates the growth of new ones. You force

the body to re-grow or repair old and damaged capillaries.

THE LYMPHATIC SYSTEM

The main function of the lymphatic system is to remove *interstitial* fluid—the fluid that bathes and surrounds cell tissue. On average, 16 percent of our total body weight is composed of interstitial fluid. To circulate this fluid, there need be a constant influx of fluid *from the capillaries*. The lymphatic system removes excess fluid and eventually returns this to the blood system via the lymphatic ducts, to one of the two subclavian (serving the neck and arm on the left or right side of the body) veins. If the removal of interstitial fluid is not functioning properly, a buildup will cause an edema (excess watery fluid in the cavities or tissues of the body).

The lymphatic system also absorbs and transports fatty acids and chyle ("a milky fluid consisting of fat droplets and lymph. It drains from the lacteals of the small intestine into the lymphatic system during digestion"). It also transports white blood cell between the lymph system and bone-marrow, and transports antibody-presenting cells to the corresponding lymph node where an immune response is activated.

The *thymus* is the primary lymphoid organ and is where maturation of T-cells occurs. The spleen is also an important part of the lymph system, responsible for regulating the immune system and blood cells. The tonsils and the thymus are also counted as part of our lymphatic system.

LYMPHATIC SYSTEM

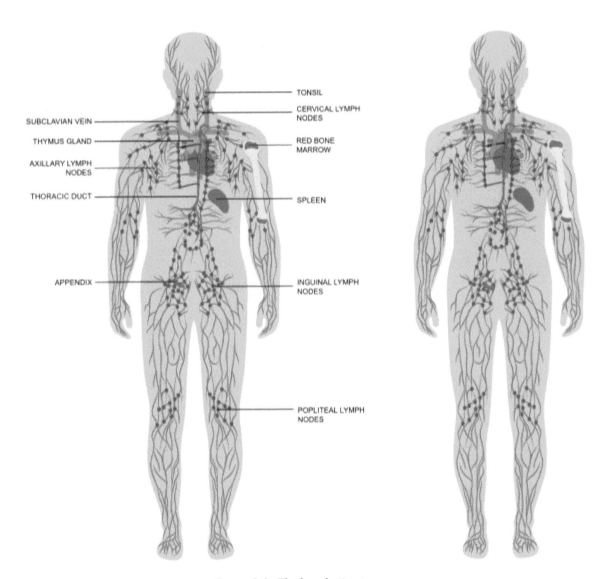

Image 1-2: The lymphatic stsyem

We each have between 500 and 600 lymph nodes in our bodies, where lymph passes through on the way back to the blood system. Lymph nodes play an important role in the regulation of the immune system. Lymph capillaries drain into lymph vessels, or *lymphatics*, which transport lymph fluid distally to centrally. The active structure in a lymph vessel is called a *lymphangion*—the segment between two valves—which performs a contractile function, mimicking a mechanical pump. Lymph is also transported through compressional force, generated by muscle activity and movement.

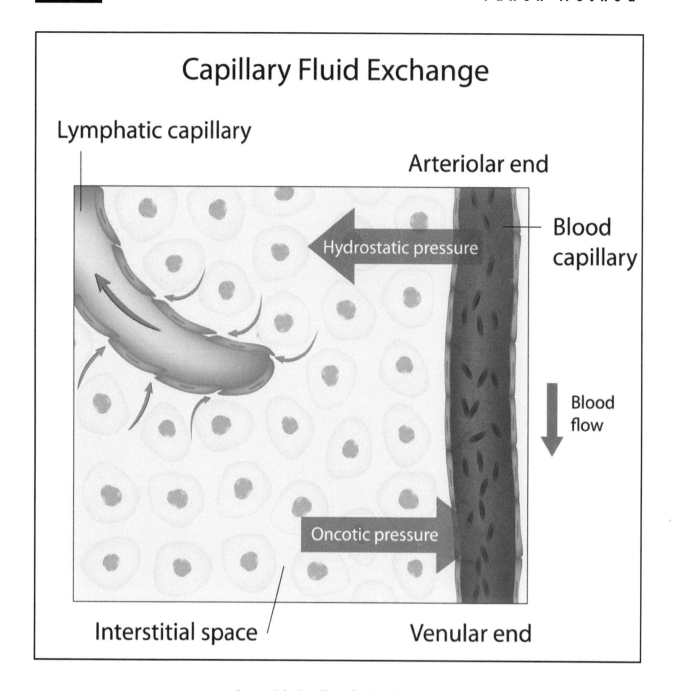

Image 1-3: Capillary fluid exchange

The circulatory system and the lymphatic system are connected by the capillary bed. A reduced circulation system usually leads to reduced lymph transportation. Signs and symptoms of decreased function of the lymphatic system include edema in arms and/or legs.

[2] BRUISING

Why do patients bruise, and why is this vital for getting optimal results?

What body structures and functions are we affecting with the Tuxen Method?

Using the Tuxen Method we create bruises with the vacuum cup. The smallest blood vessels—the capillaries—suffer microscopic tears when you apply the vacuum cup. The bruise itself is the blood that has thus permeated through the small capillary tears, not very different from a bruise on your shin when you accidentally hit your leg.

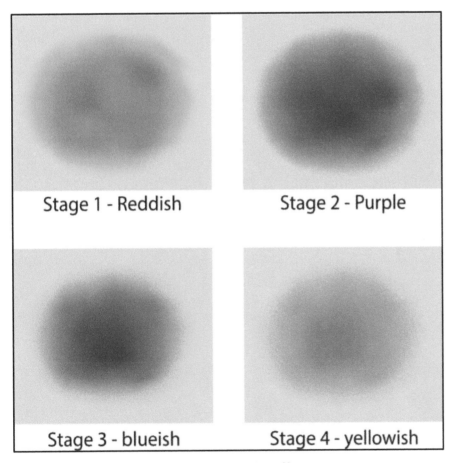

Stage 1 - Reddish

Stage 2 - Purple

Stage 3 - blueish

Stage 4 - yellowish

When you have created a bruise, the body will go through *four* different stages in the healing process, and the process normally takes between two to four days to heal, depending on the degree of bleeding (of the capillaries), circulatory condition, and the general health of the patient. The average time to heal a medium to large bruise is about one week. It is not advised to repeat the treatment before the coloring has vanished.

Image 2-1: Stages 1-4 of bruising.

- Stage 1: Bruise is fresh, appears reddish due to the color of blood leaked from the capillaries under the skin;

- Stage 2: Often after 1-2 days, but can also happen immediately. Bluish or purple color. Bluish because the blood cells (hemoglobin) have ceased transporting oxygen;

- Stage 3: Greenish color, hemoglobin breakdown, and tissue regeneration (often after 4-6 days);

- Stage 4: Yellow or brown color, usually after 4-10 days. In this stage the body absorbs the blood.

There are three main kinds of blood vessels:

1. Arteries

2. Veins

3. Capillaries

When the blood is pumped out of your heart, it enters your arteries, and is distributed through a complex system of different vessels, and finally flows into the capillaries. Capillaries are like bridges between your arteries and veins. They are so tiny that you can't see them without a microscope. The role of capillaries is to transport blood from the arteries and veins to every corner of the body and into muscles. The capillaries trade nutrition and oxygen for waste materials.

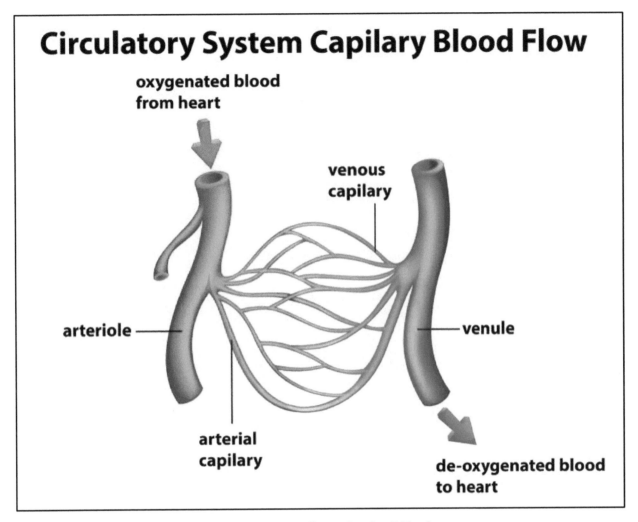

Image 2-2: Capillaries "trading" blood.

You want to have a healthy and well-functioning capillary system where the capillaries function at their optimal level. The circulatory system functions optimally at a young age. A younger person regenerates tissue damage rapidly compared to an older person if they cut themselves, for example. An older person with co-morbidity such as heart problems, high blood pressure and diabetes, will require a prolonged period of regeneration compared to a younger person if they suffer an identical injury.

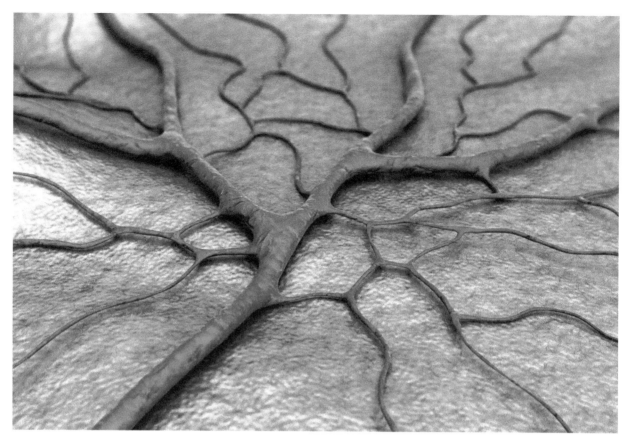

Image 2-3: Illustration of capillary system.

WHY IS BRUISING IMPORTANT?

Capillary re-growth can happen in two ways:

1. Through exercise, which challenges the circulatory system and causes a physical adaptation to a higher density of capillaries, or

2. Through conventional cell mitosis, where old cells are replaced with new ones.

Using the Tuxen Method we create microscopic tears of the capillary wall, forcing regeneration of the capillary system, thereby replacing old cells with new. This will cause an improvement in the circulatory capabilities of the treated area. In our experience, more bruising occurs in areas where the patient has complaints. It is unknown why this is so, but over- and underuse of muscles surrounding the area could perhaps be one explanation. If an area has decreased capillary function, this would diminish the exchange of nutrients as well as oxygen and carbon dioxide, and thereby render a decreased overall function in that area of the body.

In principle, Tuxen Method is analogous to strength training, where microscopic tears in muscle causes a beneficial adaptation—you break down the "old" muscle to force the body to rebuild a stronger, "new" muscle. Breaking down tissue is a common concept within physical therapy. Numerous soft-tissue techniques exist that cause this effect, including shockwave therapy, needling, massage, foam-roller, and more.

We believe the Tuxen Method excels in treating the capillary system. The vacuum provides a perfect medium to promote capillary breakdown and re-growth. Most soft-tissue techniques use a variety of compressive force. Unfortunately, compressive load is not particularly suited to promote the wanted capillary microscopic tears, as muscle and fat protect the tissue in a much more effective way during compression.

CHRONIC VERSUS ACUTE INJURY AND HEALING

It is believed that the body mobilizes in a more effective way when an acute injury occurs, as compared to a long-standing musculoskeletal problem. Why this occurs is currently unclear, but one theory is the brain concludes, in the case of long-term musculoskeletal problems, that the problem in question is not of a serious nature, and thereby decreases the focus given the region. In contrast, an acute injury causes a much larger response both circulatory and neurologically. Thus, by creating an artificially acute injury, one tries to create a larger response from the body and thereby empower faster healing.

Arteriosclerosis is a common disease where thickening, hardening, and loss of elasticity of the arterial walls cause a decrease of arterial function. The capillaries can undergo the same pathological change, and thereby compromise the transport of nutrients and exchange of oxygen and carbon dioxide. This again causes various circulatory issues, depending on the location. The Tuxen Method aims at addressing this issue on a capillary level. Note that the Tuxen Method is not a treatment for arteriosclerosis. Arteriosclerosis is just used as a metaphor to pathological changes within the capillaries.

It is also believed that tense muscles over a prolonged period of time can cause stiffness, hardening, and loss of elasticity of the capillaries. Therefore, decreased muscle tension is also a treatment goal. By application of the vacuum cup, as with other soft-tissue techniques, decreased tension of muscles can be achieved.

Pain, muscle tension, and decreased capillary function can alter movement patterns. The body is then forced to move in a suboptimal manner, causing increased stress on other tissues. This then causes a vicious cycle that ultimately leads to inactivity, pain, fear-avoidance, and loss of quality of life. Patients who are inactive, who smoke, and who keep a poor diet, are especially vulnerable to loss of capillary function.

HOW FAST DO BRUISES HEAL?

In our experience, an area of pain takes longer to heal as compared to a non-painful area of tissue, with regard to bruising. The length of time in the healing process seems to be an indication of a patient's general health, and an indication of the state of the patient's local capillary system. If a patient needs 14 days to heal a medium bruise, for example, this is an indication that the circulatory system is not optimally organized, and consequently affects the level of disposable nutrients and exchange of oxygen and carbon dioxide. A person who heals quickly, within just a few days, however, generally has a better functioning circulatory system and healthier tissue.

Empirically, when a treatment creates equally large bruises on a painful area and a non-painful area, the painful area requires a longer time to heal. Naturally, bruises occur more easily as you get older. Additionally, some medications alter the qualities of the blood—in particular, those medications that cause the blood to become thinner. Various diseases can also alter the circulatory state, such as hemophilia. Deficiencies in bioflavonoids and Vitamin C may also lead to easy bruising.

BENEFITS

After a number of Tuxen Method treatments the capillaries can be expected to have re-grown, depending of course on the patient's general health. The capillary system can then transport blood more optimally in the treated area. It is not clear whether the effects are purely due to re-growth and drainage of old capillaries, or due to an increased number of capillaries, as occurs with physical activity. Regardless, we have seen remarkable results in our practice using vacuum cupping, and welcome additional research into the area.

[3] TREATMENT STRATEGIES

It is very important to explain in advance to the patient why bruise-marks occur, and why this is an integral part of healing and recovery. It is also advised to have each patient read and sign a consent form. Treat small areas initially to monitor the reaction of the tissue in the next session. The initial treatments are usually the most painful, so also start gently. Inform the patient that they might experience slight aching after treatment, especially the day after and sometimes for up to a week. Use your own clinical judgment with regard to patient's age, circulatory state, level of physical activity, diseases, and medication with regard to dosage.

Some patients experience tiredness and aching pain, and may have a sense of exasperated symptoms after a treatment. It is therefore vital that you communicate well with your patient. In a treatment-session, inform the patient that they must give you, as the therapist, feedback with regard to pain-level. Adjust the pressure according to the feedback. Remember that more is not necessary better—in fact, you want to create microscopic tears, so start gently and listen to the patient's feedback. It is not advisable to surpass a score of 4 on a visual analog scale of pain. An optimal breakdown and healing is the treatment goal, so if too much breakdown has occurred, healing time can be unnecessary long.

We advocate use of the VAS score (Visual Analog Scale) which is a subjective feedback on pain:

- A patient rating of zero (0) would indicate the absence of pain, at one extreme, and

- A patient rating of ten (10) at the other extreme, would indicate unimaginable pain!

We recommend you share the following chart with your patient:

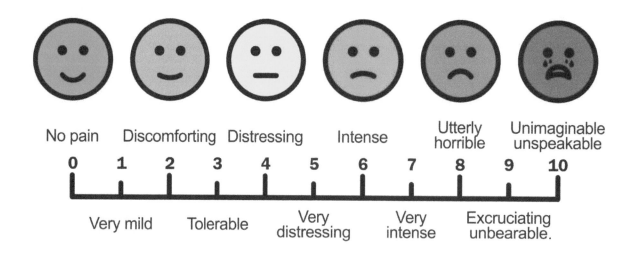

Image 3-1:VAS score

The general treatment principles are to start locally on a muscle (painful area) and then move globally. On the spine you would start centrally and then move laterally. This is because the spine is where most of the muscles attach, and where the nervous system branches out and runs to all of the muscles.

HOW TO APPLY TUXEN METHOD

If the patient remains sore a week after a treatment (even if two or three treatments into therapy), the treatment is either too aggressive or the patient might have an undiagnosed underlying issue with their health. Remember to account for all aspects that can alter the healing process:

1. Age

2. Sex

3. Level of physical fitness

4. Disease

5. Medication

6. Psychological health

7. Diet

8. Work

If the patient still has bruising when they return for their next session, it is inadvisable to treat the same area(s), as the tissue is still in the regenerative phase. Wait until the bruises are completely gone before treating the area again. Most people, however, are ready for additional treatments in the same areas after one week (seven days), while some will need up to 14 days to properly heal (and bruising disappears).

If there is no effect or apparent progress after five (5) treatments, then the Tuxen Method is probably not the correct treatment at the moment. Other things likely need to be addressed for the patient's progress, at least initially.

Don't over-treat your patients!

CAN PATIENTS BECOME SYMPTOM-FREE?

Yes, of course they can, and this is the main goal for the treatment. But as with any other treatment, this must take into account the patient's whole life, as the patient's general health and even life situations will affect treatment results. It is therefore important and advised that you inform your patients that they can contribute to optimal results by taking personal responsibility for their level of physical activity, mental well-being, and their diet.

[4] HOW GENERAL HEALTH AFFECTS TREATMENT

NEGATIVE FACTORS

There are positive and negative factors that will affect treatment outcomes. The negative factors that may influence treatment include:

- Stress

- Smoking

- Obesity

- Inactivity

- Diseases

- Medication

- Diet

- Psychological health

- Work (usually regarded as a negative factor)

POSITIVE FACTORS

Factors that may influence treatment positively include:

- Enough sleep

- Exercise

- Healthy diet

- Low intake of sugar

- Good balance between omega 3/6

- Enough Vitamin D

- Meditation/reduction of stress

- Clean water and air

- Positive personal relationships

- Positive perceived work environment

- Supplements (if indicated)

REACHING "PLATEAU"

When treated areas no longer bruise, the tissue has probably re-grown a healthy system of capillaries, and there is no longer much gain to be had from further treatment in that particular area of the body for the time being. However, if the patient still has some pain or loss of function, a different area should be treated. Remember that the body works in a complex system to provide the functions required. Sometimes several areas have to be targeted before lasting results occur.

Communicate this to you patients, and together develop an extended treatment plan. Refer your patient to other health professionals if you suspect examinations or treatment that you do not provide can offer further assistance and progress.

[5] CONTRAINDICATIONS AND WHEN TO TREAT WITH CAUTION

CONTRAINDICATIONS

Cancer: Never treat an area with cancerous tissue, however even with patients who have cancer, areas of the body with no cancer can be treated, depending on the type of cancer. Confer with a medical doctor if in doubt. Do not treat patients undergoing chemotherapy or radiation treatment.

Open wounds: Never do vacuum therapy over open wounds. Operation scars need to heal at least three months before treatment.

Genital area: Never use the vacuum machine directly on the genital area.

Tattoos: Tattoos need at least six to eight weeks to heal before performing vacuum treatment. Treat a tattoo like a minor injury of the skin, as it requires sufficient time to heal.

Pregnancy: Avoid treating pregnant women the first trimester. This is because of the general alteration of the circulatory system caused by vacuum therapy (if performed over a large area).

Additionally, 10-30% of pregnancies end up in miscarriage, and 97% of these occur within the first three months. Furthermore, take care in treating pregnant women in the last stage of pregnancy.

When in the sun: The patient should be encouraged use sun block lotion over a fresh bruise if they are to be exposed to the sun.

Contagious diseases: Do not treat patients with contagious diseases.

Infection: Do not treat infected areas.

Venous thrombosis: Circulatory diseases like deep venous thrombosis (DVT). The most common area of occurrence is in the calves, but it may appear anywhere.

WHEN TO TREAT WITH CAUTION

Loss of sensation: Any condition that inhibits sensory feedback, as this will affect the patient's ability to communicate the perceived pain level. Examples of this are nerve damage due to a trauma to a peripheral nerve, sensory loss after disc rupture, and spinal cord injuries. Treat with caution and start with low dosage.

Anticoagulant medication: Also called blood thinners or anti-platelets drugs, these drugs have various anticoagulant powers. Consult a medical doctor before prescribing vacuum therapy.

Painkillers: Drugs that alter pain-signaling may potentially decrease the patient's subjective perceived pain during treatment. As feedback from the patient is vital during vacuum therapy, painkillers may inhibit the pain response, therefore decreasing the clinical value of feedback. Treat with caution, and note which drug the patients are prescribed.

Diabetics: Treat diabetics with caution, especially around the area of insulin injections. Insulin may be stored in the tissue and be released in uncontrolled dosages if you do hard vacuum therapy over the area. However, diabetics may show significant improvement from vacuum therapy. Diabetics often have issues with poor circulation and suboptimal capillary systems. The healing process with diabetics tends to be slower and diabetics may need longer to recover from treatment. Start by treating smaller areas and with gentler treatment.

Stroke: Patients with previous stroke(s) should be treated with caution. Stroke has two main subgroups: *ischemic* and *hemorrhagic*:

- Ischemic stroke is usually caused by a thrombosis (blood-clot forming locally), or emboli (blood-clot forming somewhere in the body).

- Hemorrhagic is a bleeding in the brain itself. The altered firing from neurons in the brain that usually causes either an increase or decreased muscle-tone cannot be changed with vacuum therapy, but these patients often have muscle pain from affected areas and compensatory muscles.

Start gently and see how these patients react.

High blood pressure: When treating patients with high blood pressure there is a risk of raising the blood pressure even higher, at least temporarily, after treatment. We are not sure why, but we theorize that it could be due to changes in the capillary system and/or altered muscle tone. Areas that can affect a rise in blood pressure the most include the neck area and around the throat and head. Watch for dizziness when a patient rises from the treatment bench, as this can decrease the blood pressure momentarily.

Inflammation: Inflammation can arise from numerous causes, and it is beyond the scope of this book to cover everything related to inflammation, however we have included the most common inflammatory states seen in a clinical practice:

- If there is an active inflammation and the area is warm, swollen, and red, it is not advised to perform vacuum therapy. If you suspect a bacterial infection (note that *infection* is not the same as *inflammation*, although infection usually causes an inflammation), inform the patient that he or she should consult a medical doctor.

- Inflammation in a joint due to a rheumatological disease should not be treated when it is in an active phase. These should be referred to a medical doctor.

- A post-exercise inflammation can be treated once the acute phase has subsided. Start gently and use clinical judgment.

Chronic disease: Patients that suffer from a chronic disease often have a reduced circulatory and altered homeostatic state, and may require longer recovery periods after each treatment session. Consult a medical doctor if you are unsure if vacuum therapy is contra-indicated. If vacuum therapy is indicated, start treatment gently with fewer areas to ensure sufficient recovery after each treatment.

Areas where large arteries and veins pass: Be cautious with any area where large veins and arteries pass (see image below):

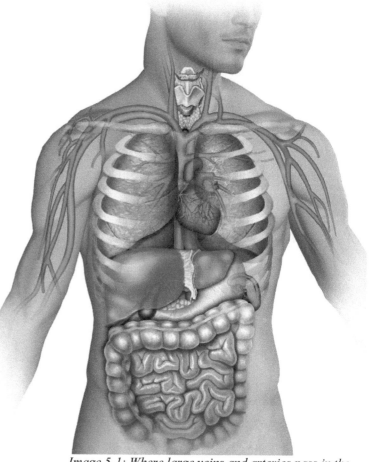

Image 5-1: Where large veins and arteries pass in the upper body

- Throat (large veins and arteries pass/cross superficially, and the area is sensitive psychologically)

- Armpit (sensitive skin, veins and arteries)

- Chest (sensitive skin and sensitive area psychologically)

- Groin area (large arteries and veins, and sensitive skin)

- Stomach area (sensitive area, close to various organs)

- Ribcage frontal (sensitive area)

- Head (sensitive area)

- Cervical area (the dorsal part of the cervical area can usually be treated with higher intensity than the lateral part)

- Face (sensitive skin, especially infraorbital margin [below the eyes])

Psychological disorders: This is a large subject, far beyond the scope of this book. However, use your clinical judgment when accepting patients with a psychological disease. There is a vast range of severity, from depression to schizophrenia. Usually, however, you can treat patients with mild psychological disorders. Consult with a medical doctor if unsure. Start gently.

The elderly patient: Ensure you uncover any comorbidity (diseases that co-occur) in the anamnesis (patient's account of their own medical history), as elderly patients statistically have a higher risk of diseases, which in turn may affect treatment. Also, pay attention to prescribed drugs as some of these may influence treatment.

Generally the recovery process slows with increased age, so longer intervals between sessions is advised. Bruises may persist longer, and decreased elasticity in the skin suggests milder treatments. In these cases, do not treat several areas in one session. Focus on the area where their main problem is located instead.

Treating children: Anamnesis with children can be challenging, as their ability to express pain and loss of function is not fully developed. Communicate well with parents and together develop a treatment plan. Beware of typical pediatric disorders like Sever's disease, osteochondritis dissicans, Osgood Schlatter disease, Legg-Calvé-Perthes disease (LCPD), and juvenile arthritis. Consult a pediatrician if unsure.

Children usually don't have circulatory issues, but may suffer from muscle aches and injuries. In our experience, one cannot palpate muscle tension in children as easily as with older patients.

Children usually respond faster to treatment, but treat gently. There is no need to produce bruises as the capillary system is usually functioning well. Never treat children with a high intensity of pain, and always cooperate with the parents. Do not treat children under four years of age. Gentle massage is often more applicable.

The sensitive patient: Although not considered a medical diagnosis, some patients tend to have a more sensitized global response than others, due to unknown causes. The sensitive patient often has a sensitive skin and pain response. Usually, they have a history of various issues. Typical diseases include Chronic Fatigue Syndrome (CFS) or fibromyalgia. These patients often suffer from minor psychological problems and chronic pain. Exercise seems to exacerbate their symptoms and they typically need longer recovery periods. Even a gentle touch can elicit pain, and they often get a strong reaction to gentle stimulation. They may also respond with tiredness and exhaustion, and typically recover more slowly.

Treat these patients very gently. As they usually improve more slowly, be patient and communicate with them about this. In most cases, the nervous system adapts to the treatment, enabling more intensive treatment at a later stage in the treatment period. Be sure to consult with other health professionals such as medical doctors, psychologists, and dietitians, when indicated.

[6] PAIN

Pain is defined by the International Association for the Study of Pain as: "An unpleasant sensory and emotional experience associated with actual or potential tissue damage, or described in terms of such damage." To give an accurate explanation of pain is a tedious and never-ending story, as the research continues to evolve. However, we will try to compound recent, up-to-date knowledge in this chapter.

Previously, the degree of pain was considered an accurate measure of tissue damage. This is no longer so. Consider athletes that break their leg, apparently with no pain-sensation over the ensuing seconds as their brain processes the damage. Only then does the athlete experience pain.

So, what is really going on neurologically? In most tissue, we have what is now called "danger" receptors (note that it is no longer referred to as nociceptors). These are C-fibers and A-delta-fibers. These fire when stimulated by various mediators, and send a signal up to the central nervous system (CNS). At this time, it is only a signal, not pain. At corresponding levels in the CNS, signals are filtered, meaning a certain number of fibers have to fire in order to send the signal further up the spine towards the brain. On the way to the frontal lobe of the brain, where it is believed the experience of pain originates, it passes through the limbic system.

The limbic system modifies the signal in a peculiar manner. It is known that depression boosts the signal, while happiness decreases it. Furthermore, prolonged stress has a tendency to increase the signal, while sudden stress that triggers the fight-or-flight response, decreases it.

When the modified "danger" signal finally reaches the frontal lobe, the brain does an overall judgment as to whether this signal is worthy of a pain-signal. To do this it summarizes all compiled knowledge including memory, emotions, culture, social, cognitive, and beliefs. Imagine a small child that only starts to cry after he or she sees blood. This is the brain processing information about the injury, and uses previous knowledge that blood indicates a larger extent of tissue injury.

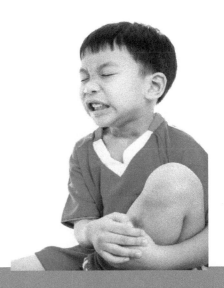

In a clinical setting this complicates matters. One should always try to get an overall picture of all contributing factors that drive each particular person's pain, and address these if possible. If it is outside your professional boundary, refer them to the correct discipline to aid your treatment.

CUPPING TECHNIQUE

[7] MANUAL CUPPING VERSUS CUPPING WITH A MACHINE

There are several benefits of investing in a professional cupping vacuum machine:

- You are able to treat several areas of the body in one session,

- You can prescribe more intense treatments,

- The strain on *you* as a massage therapist is considerably less,

- And our impression is that generally, the results are better.

The machine will provide continuous vacuum, enabling more dynamic and flexible techniques, as you don't have to remove the cup to generate vacuum manually.

You are capable of more precision and consistent suction on the treated area—even on the hair-covered areas. The cup will not slip as easily, making the treatment more efficient. Treating the ventral (underside) of the leg over the tibialis anterior, for example, or the plantar (sole) of the foot, is much easier with a machine. This is very difficult with manual cups, as they are not able to create the necessary vacuum required over these areas.

Manual cups may be used for a mild treatment, however, and are cheaper to purchase. If cupping is a new modality for you as a therapist, they may serve as an entrance to the world of vacuum therapy. You'll soon discover however, that the issues mentioned above limit your effectiveness.

THE TUXEN MACHINE

In our own practice, we invested in our own design and manufactured machine. We found that the commercially available machines were not strong enough for all treatment challenges such as plantar

facia problems, shin splints, treating the head (and other areas with a lot of hair), fingers and toes, facelifts, blackheads, and so on.

For more information about the Tuxen Method proprietary machine and how to obtain your own please visit our website www.tuxenmethod.com.

CLEANING THE CUPS

The cups must be cleaned between every patient, both for hygienic and practical reasons. The cups are best cleaned using warm water and normal dishwashing solution since this dissolves fatty substances effectively. Use protective gloves for hygiene and to protect your skin. Apply an antibacterial solution after drying.

The rubber suction-ball will harden on manual cups over time, so replace when appropriate.

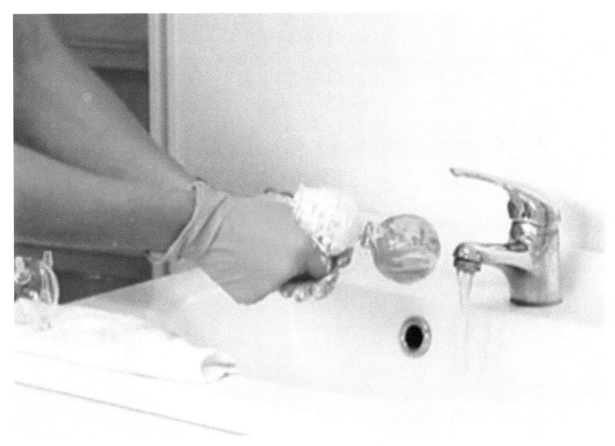

Image 7-1: Cleaning a manual cup

[8] CUPPING TECHNIQUES FOR MUSCLES

Y ou can move the cups in all directions, and vary the pressure from high to low. You can also change between small and big cups for different intensities. A small cup will have a higher vacuum force versus a larger one, with the same suction-power of the machine. You can also vary between short and long strokes for different results. In the pages and images that follow we will demonstrate some of the most common therapeutic techniques with cups.

THE MOST COMMON TECHNIQUES

Working across the muscle (medially to laterally and laterally to medially)

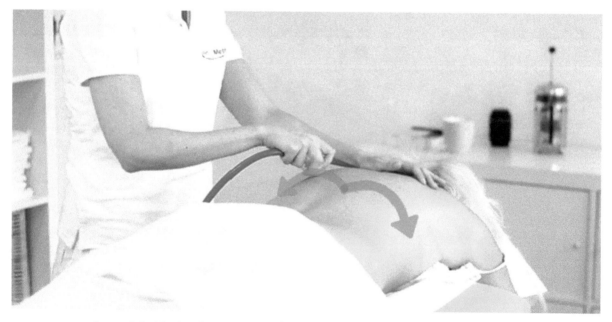

Image 8-1: Moving the cup across the muscle medially to laterally and vice versa

Working longitudinal (across the muscle fibers and reverse)

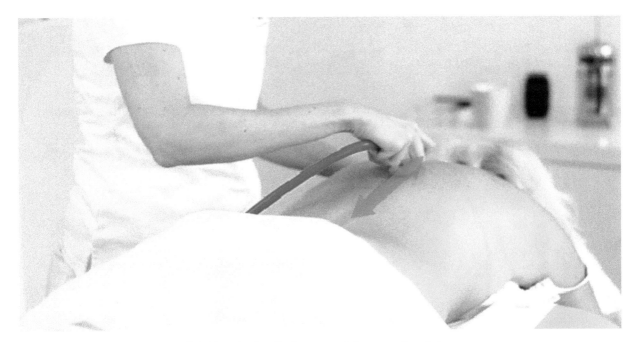

Image 8-2: Longitudinally from cranial to sacral and vice versa.

Working oblique

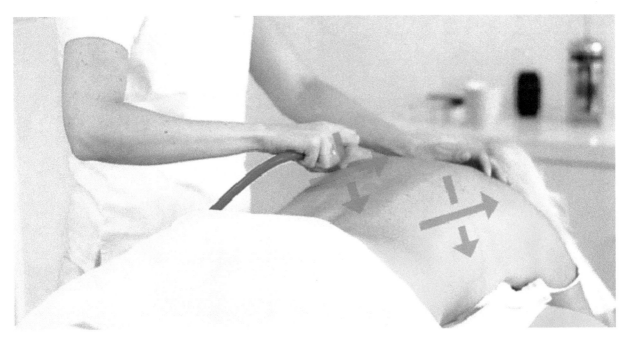

Image 8-3: Moving the cup obliquely. Do this in opposite directions making a cross over the treatment area to release tension in the muscle and stretch the fascia.

Circular work

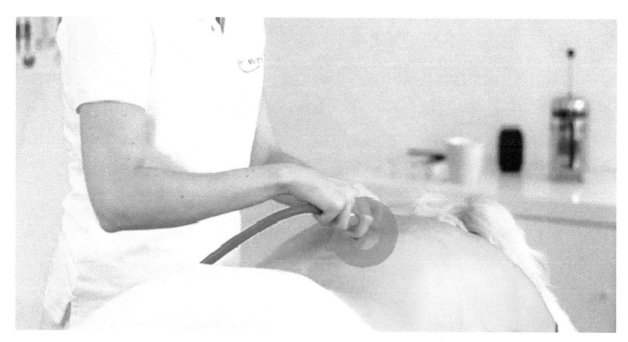

Image 8-4: The cups being moved in circles.

Trigger point work

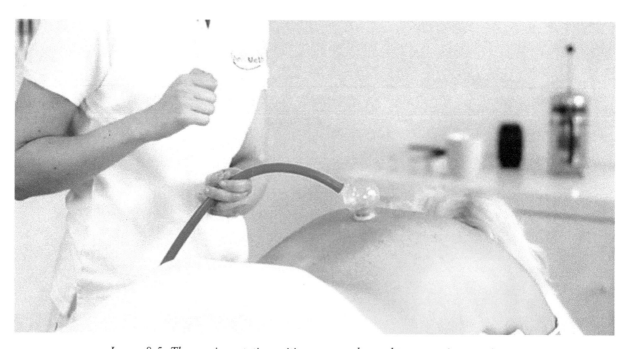

Image 8-5: The cup in a static position commonly used to treat trigger points.

Working with muscle in resting position

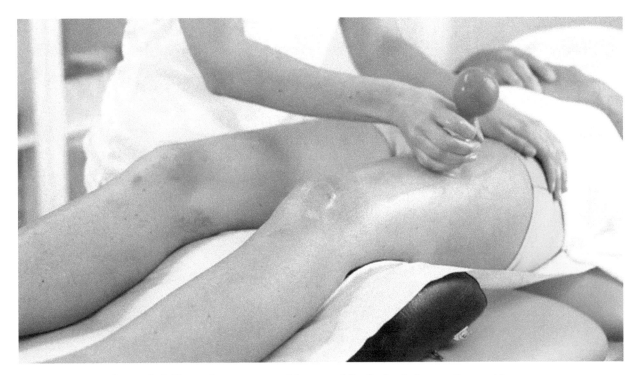

Image 8-6: Dynamic movement of the cup while the leg is in a resting position.

Working in stretched position

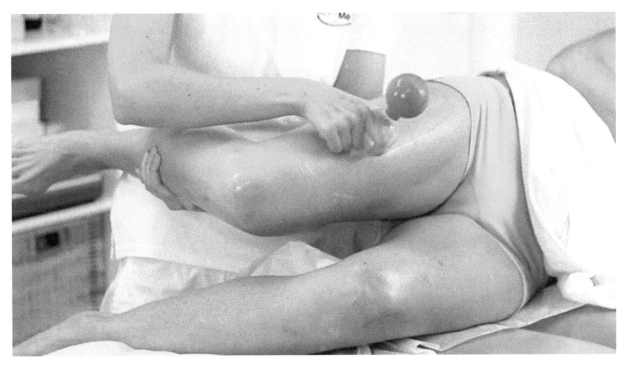

Image 8-7: Dynamic movement of the cup while the muscle is in a stretched position.

Tuxen Method with **active dynamic movement**

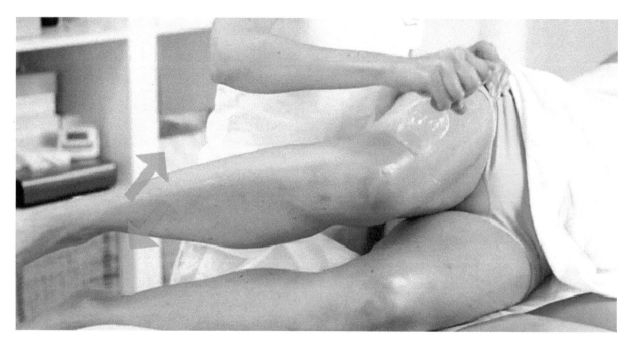

Image 8-8: Active movement with dynamic movement of the cup

Tuxen Method with **isometric movement**

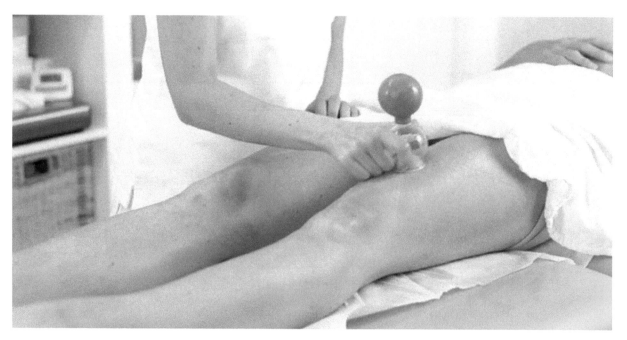

Image 8-9: Static position of cup while doing isometric movement (activating and relaxing the muscle)

Tuxen Method for **deep tissue massage effect**

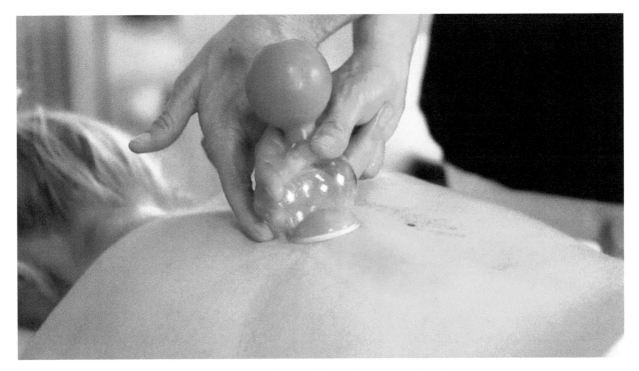

Image 8-10: The cup in static position, with small tilt to one side for more intensity.

Every technique can be either aggressive or gentle, depending on the amount of vacuum generated. This can be adjusted on the vacuum machine, and by the size of the cup as well. Intensity will also vary depending on use of short or long strokes, and speed of the movement.

GENERAL APPLICATION TIPS

- Less aggressive longitudinally with the muscle fibers.

- More aggressive perpendicular to the muscle fibers.

- Less aggressive medially to laterally.

- More aggressive laterally to medially.

- With trigger points, vary the intensity with vacuum pressure and cup size.

- Small cups provide higher intensity, large cups create lower intensity.

- Small strokes create higher intensity.

- Vary static position with dynamic. For example, pause for 5-10 seconds on a position, and then assume dynamic treatment.

- Treating muscle in a resting position is less aggressive, but generates a deeper effect.

- Isometric contraction with treatment: medium aggressive, depending on the intensity and area.

- Dynamic movement with treatment is more aggressive.

- You have applied adequate treatment when either/or:

  - a bruise develops,

  - a reddish color appears in the skin,

  - or the patient's tolerance for pain is reached.

- Generally it is better to treat small areas with gentle techniques the first session.

- Develop a knowledge of how a patient's tissue tolerates treatment and develop a degree of trust with a patient before applying more aggressive techniques.

- The patient's general health and pain limit are the two most important factors in determining which treatment technique(s) you should apply.

- Attempt a more aggressive technique if the effects of treatment seem to plateau, as long as the patient can tolerate it such technique(s).

- Low intensity techniques penetrate more superficially into the muscle.

- High intensity techniques penetrate deeper into the muscle.

[9] CUPPING FOR THE FASCIAL SLINGS

The *fascia* is the biological fabric that holds us together. It is composed of fibrous connective tissue and has a multitude of functions. Fascia is divided into the *superficial*, *deep*, and the *visceral*:

- The **superficial** strata is located in the subcutis, just below the surface of the skin, blending with parts of the dermis.

- The **deep** layer surrounds, supports, and stabilizes muscles, and sometimes acts as a tendinous structure (as with tensor fascia lata and plantar fascia).

- The **visceral** layer encloses and suspends various organs.

Understanding fascia is essential to understanding stability and movement. The fascia interconnects the tendons and muscles and keeps all the organs in their correct places. The fascia aids us in functioning in a tridimensional manner and helps the muscles work smoothly together.

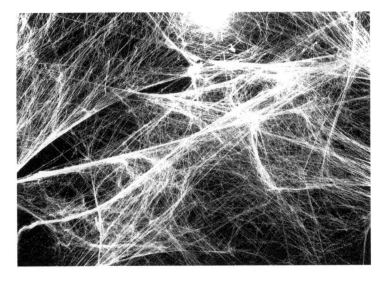

Image 9-1: The fascia has a similar structure to a cobweb.

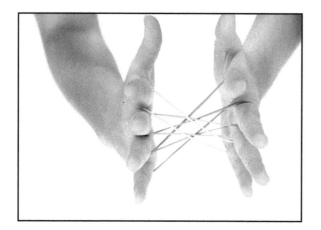

Image 9-2: Flexibility of the fascia is important.

By applying the Tuxen Method, you can target some of the superficial and deep fascias. And while it is not yet established if in doing so you physically lengthen the fascia, you very likely make it more adaptable to movement and more flexible.

With the Tuxen Method, we try to address not only one fascia, but the entire *sling* (slings are demonstrated below). Humans tend to use a combination of several joints and muscles in accomplishing a given physical task. If your examination of your patient demonstrates a lack of fascial mobility, in our experience best results are achieved when you target the entire fascial sling.

FASCIA SLINGS

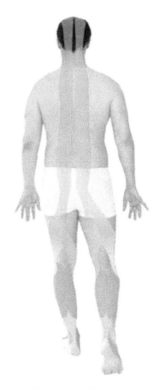

Image 9-3: Superficial back line

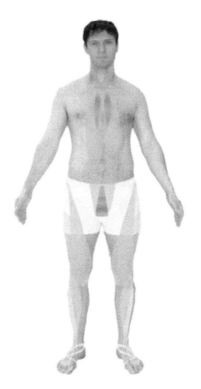

Image 9-4: Superficial front line

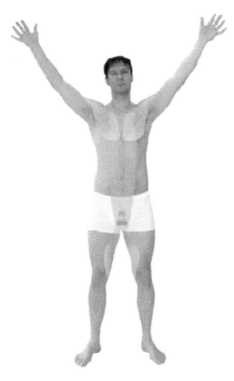

Image 9-5: Functional front line

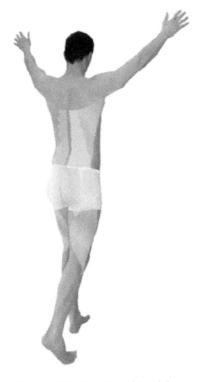

Image 9-6: Functional back line

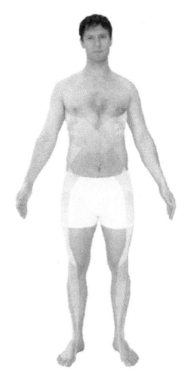

Image 9-7: The spiral line

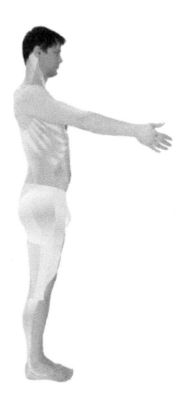

Image 9-8: The lateral line

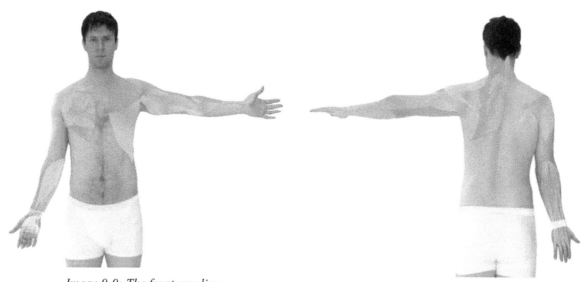

Image 9-9: The front arm line

Image 9-10: The back arm line

Example:

Painful area	Main sling	Secondary sling	Tertiary sling
Neck	Superficial	Back Arm Line	Lateral
Hamstring	Post. superficial	Lateral	Frontal

You apply this knowledge in therapy by assessing the mobility of the most relevant fascia line first. Treat this according to previously mentioned algorithm in Chapter 8 (regarding fascia). Reassess the next session. Progress to for example treating the main and the secondary. And so on. You can obviously combine this with treatments aimed at various muscles if your clinical assessment demonstrates a muscle component to the problem.

In our experience, it is advantageous to complement the treatment of fascia with various stretching exercises for the same fascial sling that you decided to treat.

[10] CUPPING TO INCREASE BLOOD CIRCULATION

LOCALLY

You can always work directly and treat areas locally, but it may be beneficial to activate certain areas prior to treatment to increase the effect.

UPPER EXTREMITY

1.   Target the scalene area as well as above and below the clavicle, and the pectoralis minor area.

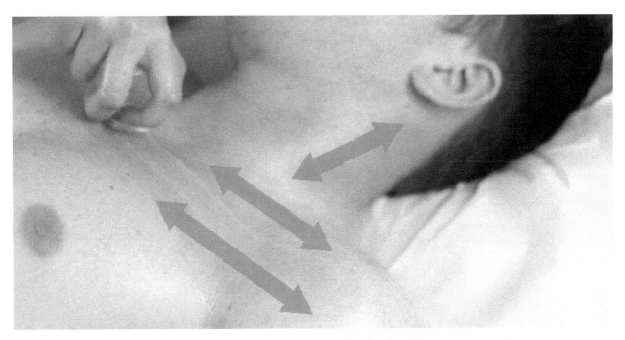

Image 10-1: Tuxen Method on the scalene-area, above/below the clavicle and the pectoralis minor area.

2. Target the diaphragm. The diaphragm surrounds the vena cava, the largest blood vessel in our body. This vein transports deoxygenated blood from the intestines and lower extremity back to the right atrium. In theory, a tight diaphragm can influence the function of the vena cava.

3. Target the intercostal muscles. You may also want to work on the whole rib cage to release tension in the intercostal muscles to help the diaphragm indirectly. By decreasing the activity of the intercostal muscles, the rib cage is allowed to expand easier. Thereby, decreasing the load on the diaphragm.

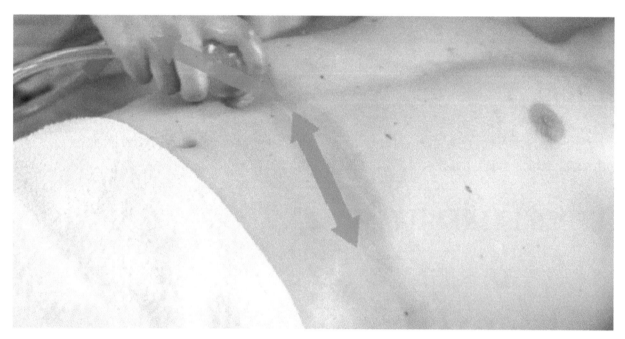

Image 10-2: Circulation treatment working directly on the diaphragm.

4. Target the forearm. Another important area for circulation for the forearm is the palmar area where the median nerve passes through the carpal tunnel. Decreased space here gives rise to Carpal Tunnel Syndrome. This is more prevalent among late-stage pregnant women, probably due to a increase of fluid.

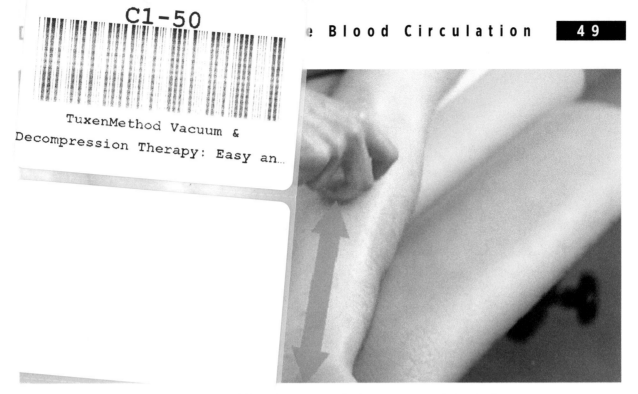

Image 10-3: Treatment of the palmar area to help increase circulation in the arm.

UNDER EXTREMITY

Treat groin area/femoral triangular.

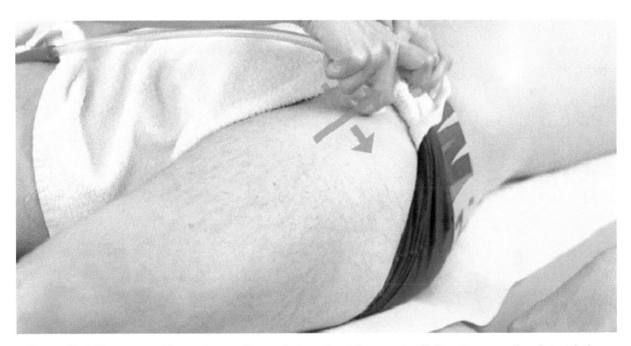

Image 10-4: Treatment of the groin area/femoral triangular. Move cup in all directions to pull and stretch the fascia in all directions.

Posterior side of knee

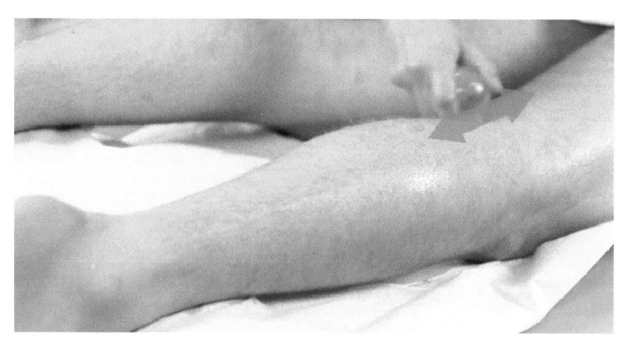

Image 10-5: Treatment of the posterior side of knee.

Posterior part of lower leg

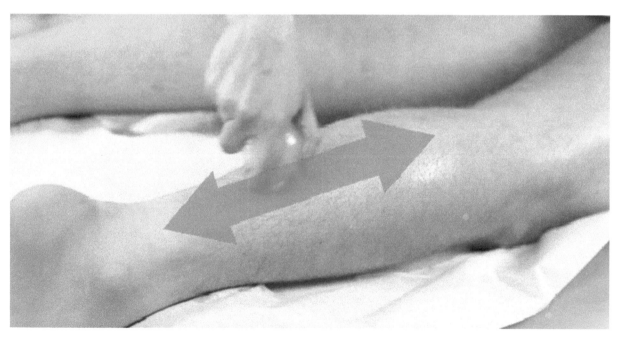

Image 10-6: Figure showing the Tuxen Method on increasing circulation in the whole leg.

Always advise patients to be physically active, to increase their heart rate to achieve maximum results in (circulation) treatment.

[11] TREATING THE LYMPH SYSTEM

There are two main ways to stimulate the lymph system with the Tuxen Method:

TREATMENT METHOD 1

The first method is to do a gentle vacuum treatment to stimulate the lymphatic flow. When applying, treat from distal/lateral to proximal/medial.

TREATMENT METHOD 2

Alternatively, use the same principles and techniques aiming to increase circulation, covered in chapter 2 and 9. The close relationship between lymphatic function and blood flow, ensures that both should be addressed for maximum effect. In our experience, Treatment Method 1 has better results on patients with a global decreased function of the lymphatic system. Treatment Method 2 is an excellent tool when patients have a local swelling. We recommend this method on, for example, post-acute (2-3 days after trauma) ankle sprains, where it can significantly decrease the swelling with only a couple of treatments.

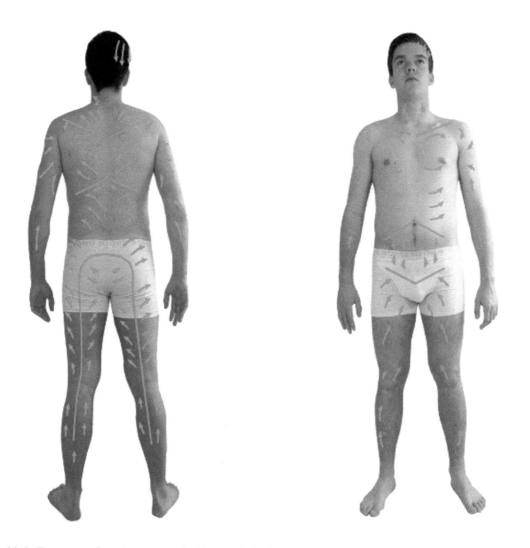

Image 11-1: Treatment directions using the Tuxen Method. Important areas are the groin and the clavicle-area.

[12] THE DIGESTIVE SYSTEM

Eighty to 90 percent of our immune system lies in the digestive system. Imbalance in the digestive system may lead to being overweight, depression, allergies, constipation, Alzheimer's disease, among other ailments and illnesses. Recent research is suggesting a direct relationship between the digestive system and the rest of the body. For example, people with irritable bowel syndrome (IBS) have a higher incidence of depression and sadness.

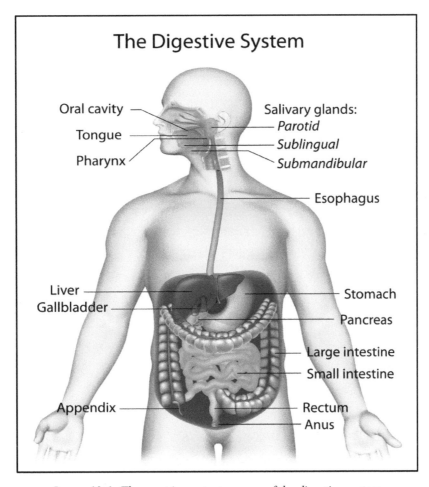

Image 12-1: The most important organs of the digestive system.

The colon is a large part of our immune system. Research shows that the inner bacterial flora in the colon might control close to 80 percent of the immune system. Stress, reduced physical activity, poor nutrition, and food intolerance can lead to a compromised digestive system, often manifesting in either constipation or diarrhea and gas pain. Stress activates the sympathetic nervous system which hampers food digestion. Activity, on the other hand, increases interstitial contraction, leading feces further down the colon. A compromised digestive system also leads to reduced nutrition uptake, again affecting cell production. A poor digestive system can also lead to general muscle ache and joint pain. For example, there is a connection between rheumatoid arthritis and Crohn's disease.

Although the Tuxen Method can aid clients with digestive problems, a healthy diet is obviously vital. Discuss this with your client, and refer to a dietician if needed. Also, physical activity is important to stimulate activity of the digestive system.

If the client has a lot of stress, fear, or anxiety in their life, this should be addressed, as psychological factors may regulate the sympathetic nervous system which may lead to poor digestion. Recommend a psychologist or appropriate professional as needed.

HOW TUXEN METHOD HELPS A COMPROMISED DIGESTIVE SYSTEM

The Tuxen Method may help the function of the digestive system. Many patients have a lot of tension, or over-activity of muscles, around their digestive system, which may inhibit function. We are not sure of the exact mechanism, but it may be that an increase in tone of muscles surrounding the digestive organs decreases their effectiveness, or it may be that an increased tone may exert compressional force on the small and large intestines. The effect may also originate from stimulating the sensory pathways of the digestive anatomical area, which again regulates the sympathetic nervous system.

Nonetheless, in our experience release around the liver and diaphragm may be effective. To clarify, it is not stimulus of the organs themselves that produce clinical change.

Additionally, release around the small and large intestines may help release gas and solidified feces.

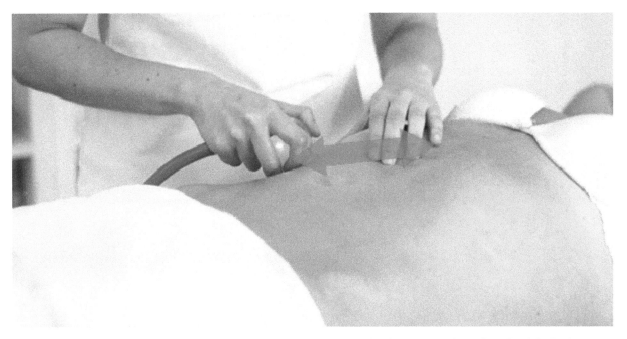

Image 12-2: How to release tension around the liver and gallbladder area on the right side of the body.

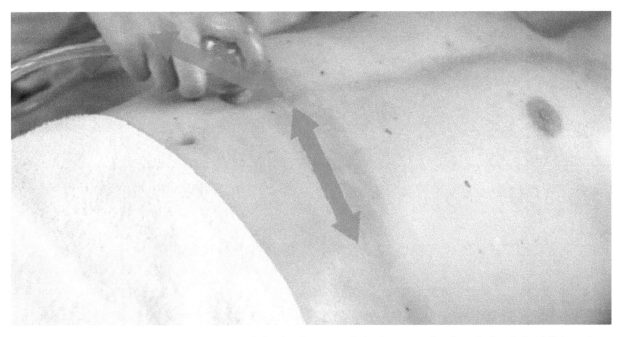

Image 12-3: How to release tension around the diaphragm to help the stomach adrenal glands (middle) and liver/gallbladder (right side) and pancreas/spleen /left side.

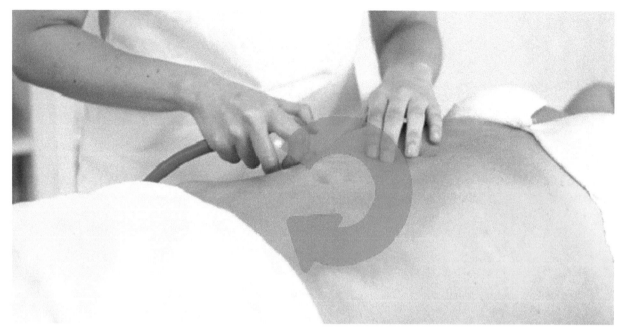

Image 12-4: How to stimulate the colon to help intestinal activity in the large intestine to help release gas and solidified feces. Work in circles in the same direction as the clock/sun.

The general rule is to follow the tension and work thoroughly around the areas with the highest tension, as these tend to be the problem areas.

THE THORACIC SPINE AND SYMPATHETIC NERVOUS SYSTEM

According to some chiropractic and osteopathic schools it is believed that you may influence all structures to their corresponding level in the spine. As for the sympathetic nervous system, it is speculated that one could generate change in various organs via muscles and the facet joints. For example, one could try to lessen the symptoms of Irritable Bowel Syndrome by treating the levels T5-7, and the vagus nerve (cranial nerve X) with the Tuxen Method.

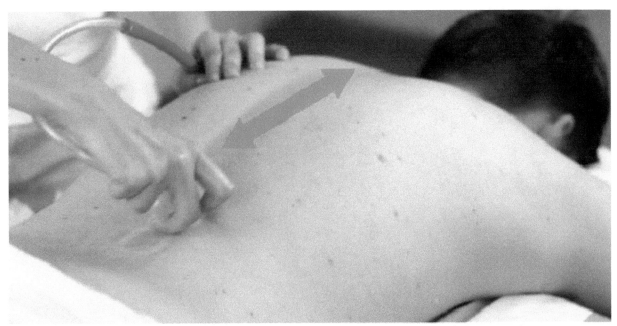

Image 12-5: The Tuxen Method stimulating the thoracic spine where the whole sympathetic nervous system runs and nerve supply to all the digestive organs emanates.

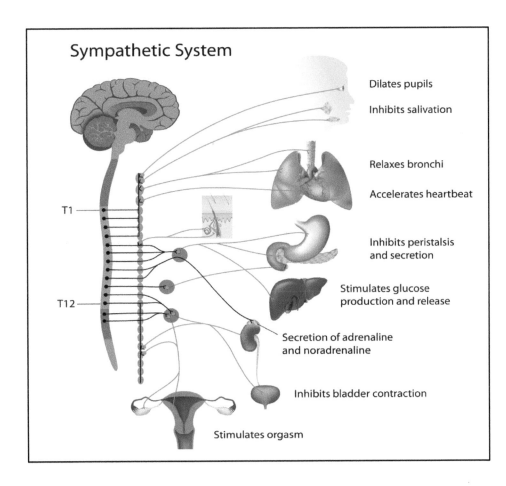

Sympathetic System

Dilates pupils

Inhibits salivation

Relaxes bronchi

Accelerates heartbeat

Inhibits peristalsis and secretion

Stimulates glucose production and release

Secretion of adrenaline and noradrenaline

Inhibits bladder contraction

Stimulates orgasm

T1

T12

Image 12-6: The thoracic spine and innervation to the various organs.

AILMENTS

[13] EMOTIONAL STRESS

Emotional stress has been found to reduce the quality of sleep, affect the immune and digestive systems, and be a risk factor for chronic pain, and people with emotional stress often experience pain in specific parts of the body. They describe symptoms like tension, heaviness, and pain. They usually don't have the same mechanical triggers of pain that arthritis of the hip may demonstrate, for example, but pain itself is often linked to a feeling or specific thought-pattern. This may be stress, fear, loneliness, depression, or any negative state. The pain is usually in an *area*, not a specific point, and behaves in a non-mechanical way. People with anxiety and depression are more prone to heart disease, stroke, and high blood pressure. In studies these people also have a shorter life expectancy than control groups.

Physical pain may also be related to emotional stress. An indication might be, for example, when someone states "Whenever I am stressed I get a headache," or "My lower back hurts when I worry." Here you get a specific indication that the emotional state leads to physical pain. Many patients are unconscious about their emotional patterns, but it still may contribute to their overall experience of pain. In such cases, emotional issues serve as the primary driver for physical pain. And it is for all accounts a physical pain, not just mechanical in nature.

If they have not consulted a psychologist or medical doctor, discuss this with the patient. The Tuxen Method can only treat the symptoms of emotional stress, not the cause, but with Tuxen Method you can, nonetheless, help the patient by decreasing the manifestation of pain.

HOW TO APPLY THE TUXEN METHOD TO ALLEVIATE STRESS

If you believe your patient may suffer from emotional stress, ask the patient where the emotional stress manifests in their body when triggered. This is obviously an individual matter, but is usually located centrally. Typical areas where emotions are often include:

- Face

- Neck

- Chest

- Stomach or gut

- Lower back

We even have everyday expressions in language which suggest where the emotion may be found, for example:

- "I have a bad feeling about this."

- "I have a heart ache."

- "I have a lump in my throat."

- "My boss is a pain in the neck."

TECHNIQUES FOR EMOTIONAL STRESS

Some patients may experience an emotional reaction during or after treatment. Inform the patient about this, and let them decide if they want to continue. You may want to encourage them to consult a psychiatrist or psychologist to treat the underlying cause of their problems.

IMPORTANT! *Do not treat patients with a personality disorder, who are emotionally unstable, or have other psychiatric diagnoses.*

Below are the most common areas that may be effective for releasing emotional stress. Ask the patient where they feel the center of their pain is and start there. Always start gently, especially the first session, and progress slowly. The focus is not to increase the circulation, but to release tension in the skin, fascia, and/or muscle.

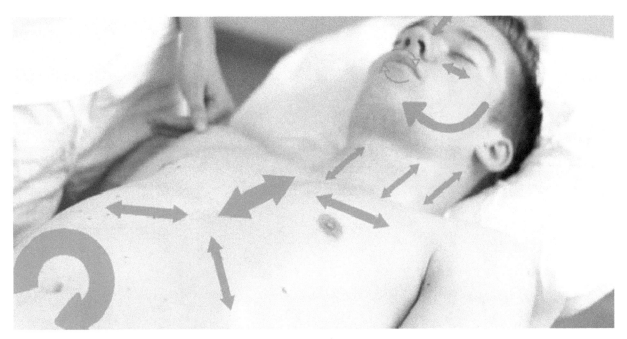

Image 13-1: Common areas with emotional pain, and direction of treatment.

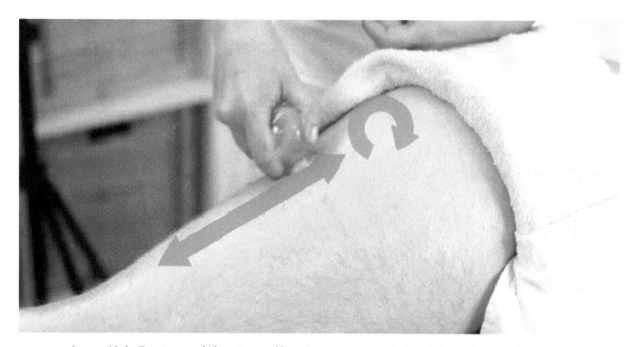

Image 13-2: Treatment of "heaviness of legs," or "no energy in legs," for a depressed patient.

[14] SINUS PROBLEMS

The Tuxen Method may be effective in decreasing symptoms associated with sinus-problems. Signs of a compromised sinus and sinus inflammation are:

- Blocked nose/congestion

- Greenish/yellow discharge

- Feeling of pressure

- Pain around face

- Headache

- Sore throat

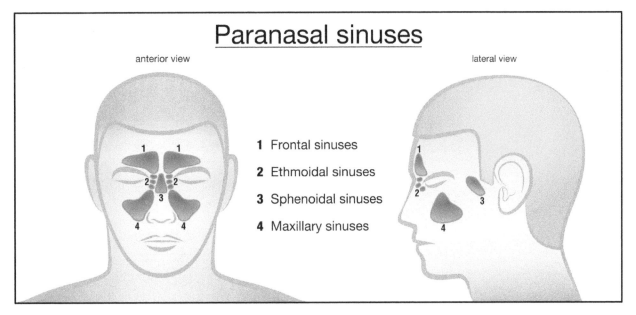

Image 14-1: The sinus channels

The Tuxen Method may help with draining of the sinus channel. The cup cannot exert vacuum in the actual sinus canal, but may stimulate drainage through stimulation of the sensory pathways, causing an alteration through the sympathetic nervous system.

In our experience, treatment of sinus problems with the Tuxen Method should be administered two times a week, and at least five times to see improvement. Start stimulating the sinus area on both sides of the head, and ask the patient where they feel the most pressure/pain. You might work dynamically or statically.

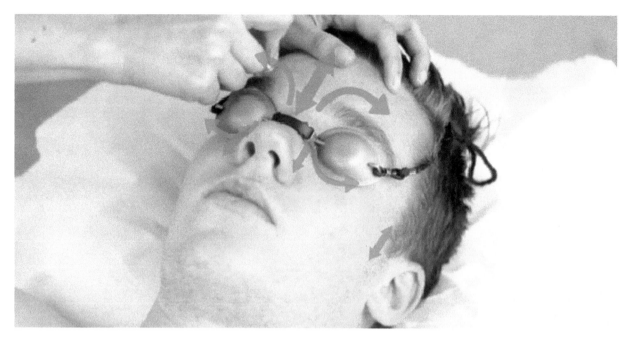

Image 14-2: *Effective areas to treat to help the draining of the sinus channel. Note plastic glasses to protect the eyes.*

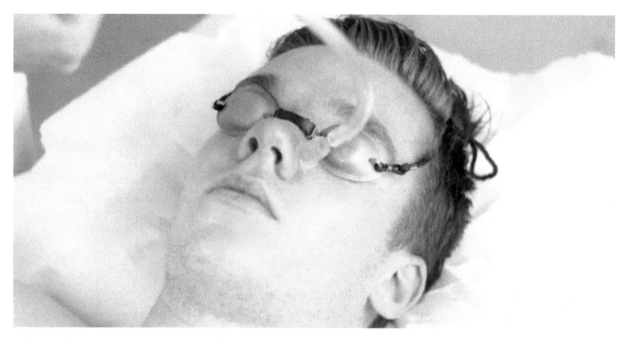

Image 14-3: *Demonstrating the use of a vacuum cup as an acupuncture needle with static technique for 10-60 seconds.*

[15] SCAR TISSUE

S car tissue is common after caesarean section and other operations and injuries. Scar tissue often decreases mobility in the skin and muscle around the area where the scar tissue is located. This can lead to either an over- or under-activity of the muscle. Often the muscle is weaker and may suffer decreased circulation.

When performing the Tuxen Method on scars, the scar should be at least be 12 weeks old, and be fully healed before treated. During the initial treatment sessions the scar may bruise quickly, but it usually heals well. You may likely need 5-10 treatments before you have achieved the maximum effect. This is occurs when there is no more bruising, even after an aggressive treatment, but the treated are appears red and well circulated.

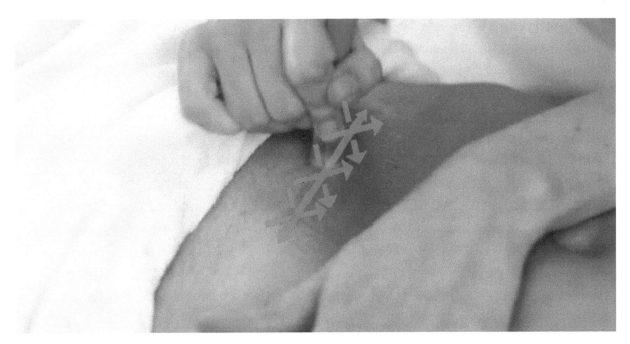

Image 15-1: Treatment of an operation scar after a cesarean. Try to pull and stretch the tissue in all directions to increase flexibility of the scar tissue. Try different Tuxen Method techniques for maximum effect

[16] VARICOSE VEINS

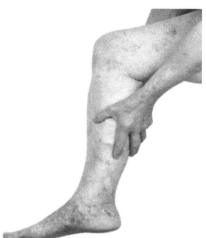

Spurred by muscle activity, blood is transported by the veins centrally by a non-return valve system. Varicose veins are caused by a defect in these valves, preventing them from closing fully. This causes the blood to flow backwards and hamper the return of the blood. This build-up of blood is believed to increase pressure within the vein, and consequently the vein increases in diameter.

Tuxen Method cannot fix the defective valves, but it can increase the circulation in general in the area and provide a drainage effect of the blood in the targeted vein. This may also decrease pain. When treating varicose veins with the Tuxen Method you generally follow the veins that you can visually see. Stimulate the area until it has a red color around the vein, or the patient feels that it is too painful to continue. Start gentle. Also advise the patient that exercise is an important part of treatment.

You can't see varicose veins in all patients, and they do vary from patient to patient as far as where the course of the vein runs and how many veins might run through the area. Combine direct treatment with more general techniques to ensure maximum results. Try to build up the vacuum gradually, as in our experience one achieves better results with more vacuum. Work up and down and across to stimulate circulation as much as possible.

NOTE: Do not mistake varicose veins for Deep Venous Thrombosis (DVT). With DVT, Tuxen Method is contraindicated, and the patients should receive medical attention as soon as possible. Also, be aware that these conditions may co-exist.

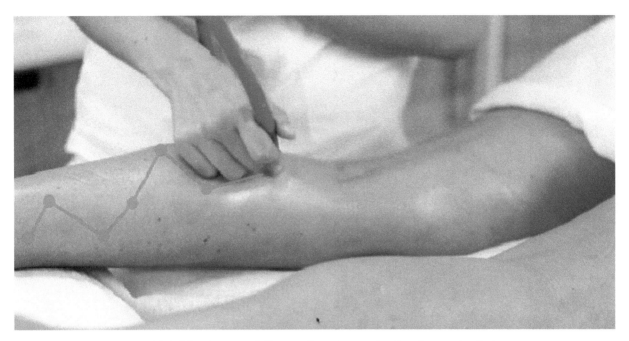

Image 16-1: The therapist following the veins to stimulate better circulation.

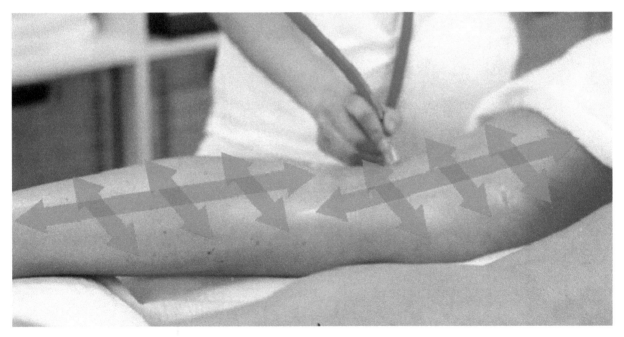

Image 16-2: The therapist applying the Tuxen Method vacuum therapy from distally to centrally along the leg, to the top of the thighs. Also, a transverse technique is used to stimulate circulation all over the leg.

[17] JOINTS

Signs and symptoms that pain is originating from the joints include:

- Pain during movement

- Morning stiffness

- Pain located in the joint

- X-ray imaging which demonstrates degenerative changes

- Reduced movement in the joint

- Swelling around the joint

All joints undergo structural changes during our lifespan, and wear and tear is inevitable. However, not all people suffer from pain from this, even if x-ray imaging shows significant changes. The definitive reason for this is yet unknown.

JOINT INJURIES

It is beyond the scope of this book to cover the vast subject of joint injuries, but keep in mind that some injuries are predominantly age-related and others are typically the result of injuries. The Tuxen Method cannot change the structure of the joint, but may modify symptoms related to the injury.

ANKLE JOINT

To stimulate the ankle joint you want to work on soleus and gastrocnemius and popliteus to increase movement in dorsi and plantar flexion. Work locally around the joint superior and inferior tibiafibular-joint to decrease tension in the muscles for better movement in the joint. This may increase supination and pronation.

KNEE JOINT

The knee joint is a common site for arthritis and acute injuries such as meniscus or cruciate ligaments. Often the knee joint will demonstrate decreased flexion and extension in a 4:1 ratio.

Work locally around the knee joint along the joint space medially and laterally. Especially check the pes anserinus-area, dorsally the popliteus, gastrocnemius and hamstring.

Also, work in a circulatory around the patella.

PATELLA

Encircle the patella with the cups gradually from one side to the other. It may be beneficial to include techniques for the quadriceps, hamstring, gastrocnemius, popliteus and soleus.

HIP JOINT

To help the patient with hip joint symptoms, target the gluteus medius/minimus/maximus, iliotibial band, dorsally of the trochanter major, psoas major/minor and iliacus. You may also want to include adductor longus/brevis, gracilis and pectineus.

FINGERS

Problems in the fingers are often either a type of arthritis or degenerative changes (often with the thumb). Fingers are also prone to acute injuries, after a fall, for example. Work over the wrist and underarm, up to the elbow, medially to laterally, and along the palmar region to help circulation and flexibility.

SHOULDER/SCAPULA

Work locally around the whole shoulder joint both anterior, lateral and posteriorly.

Anterior: deltoid, pectoralis major, pectoralis minor, anterior rotator cuff, subclavicle.

Posterior: latissimus, levator scapula, rhomboid, upper/middle/lower trapezius.

Lateral: deltoid, trapezius.

STERNO-COSTAL JOINT

Irritation in the sterno-costal joint is not uncommon. An inflammatory version of this problem is called Tietze Syndrome. Taking a deep breath, coughing, or sneezing often cause pain in the joint. Rotations of the thoracic spine may also elicit pain. The rib area may also be painful and feel stiffer when applying compression compared to the other ribs. Treat up the lines and follow the ribs front and back.

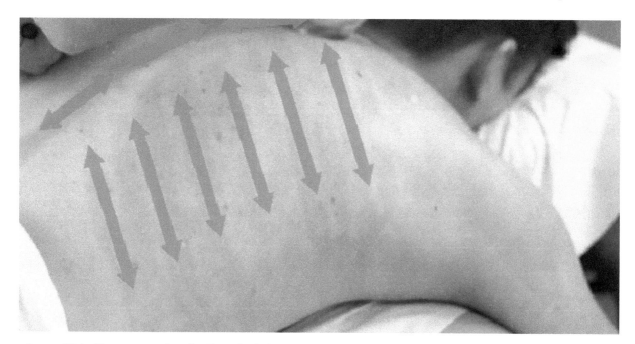

Image 17-1: How to treat the ribs. Treat both the spine and the area between the ribs. If an area is more painful you will want to spend extra time there to release the tension.

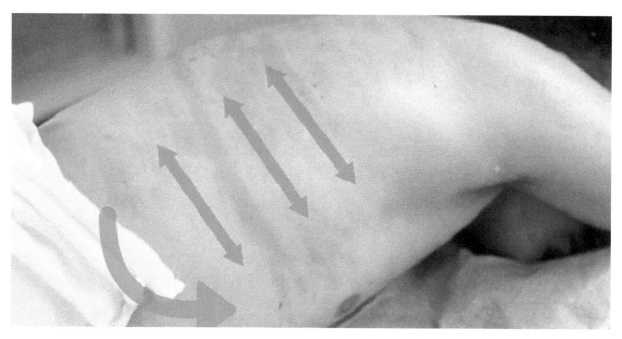

Image 17-2: How to treat the ribs. Release the diaphragm as well as the muscles between each rib.

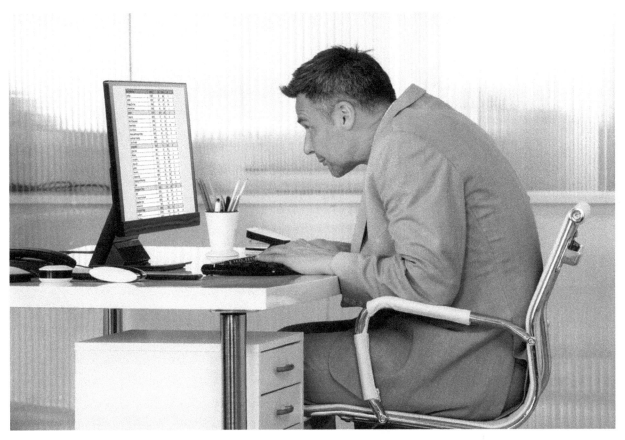

Image 17-3: An office worker sitting in a bad position for his ribs.

COSTOVERTEBRAL JOINT

Pain and loss of function where the ribs connect to the vertebra is probably less common than sterno-costal joint problems, but they do exist. Often pain in a general area over the affected joint is caused by deep inhalation, coughing or sneezing, and rotation of the trunk. Compression of the rib causes movement in the joint, and usually elicits pain.

[18] RHEUMATIC DISEASES

The term "rheumatic disease" is an umbrella term used for a variety of diseases. For simplicity, we will only address here rheumatic diseases caused by an autoimmune reaction. There are more than 200 subcategories of rheumatic diseases, so we'll also only mention the most common, and we won't go into each disease in depth, as that would be far beyond the scope of this book.

But we will focus on treatment. Obviously, the Tuxen Method cannot change the underlying process of the autoimmune disease, but we may change some symptoms of the disease. Patients suffering from rheumatic disease should be monitored and treated by a rheumatologist. The most common autoimmune rheumatic diseases are:

- Osteoarthritis

- Ankylosing Spondylitis

- Rheumatic Arthritis

- Systemic Lupus Erythematosus

- Sjogren's Syndrome

Often, patients suffering from rheumatic diseases have pain, swelling, and loss of function of various joints, depending on which subcategory of disease the patient is suffering from. They may also experience pain in muscle, bursa, and tendons.

When using the Tuxen Method, assess which structure is most associated with the current issues suffered by the patient, and treat accordingly the joint, muscle, and/or tendon. Start gently, and progress. Note that aggressive stretching of the joint and/or tendon may increase the inflammatory process. If there is no active inflammation, stretching and mobilization is considered vital in Ankylosing Spondylitis.

Rehabilitation is important in rheumatic diseases. Advise the patient to find a good physical therapist to assist your treatment. In osteoarthritis, being overweight is the most important factor, so consider referring the patient to a dietician.

[19] TENDONS

Tendons are composed of specialized connective tissue and connect muscle to bone. One of the most common complaints of musculo-skeletal injuries is called *tendinopathy*. It used to be called *tendinitis*, but this term was changed as there are only identifiable inflammatory markers in the acute stage of the condition. There may be some inflammation in a short, acute phase, but it is no longer considered a primary inflammatory condition.

Tendons can withstand substantial load, or tractional force, as a tendon is designed as a wire. It transfers force from the contracted muscle to the bone to generate movement. Too much force-transmission, with too many repetitions and not enough rest, may cause tendinopathy. A tendon will adapt to new requirements if given enough time and rest, but a large increase in load over a short period of time is not beneficial.

Gradual, gradient exposure of various exercises is considered essential to the treatment. If you are not comfortable prescribing exercises yourself, refer the patient to a physiotherapist.

Tendinopathy often causes pain in the region of the insertion, mid-portion or in the musculo-tendinous junction, and gives pain under load or compression. Tendons may be stiffer and more painful in the morning, due to increased water storage. Problems may appear at any age, but are most common in the middle-aged. With athletes tendinopathy can occur at any age, as their sport usually demands a continuous and high load.

Treatment with the Tuxen Method aims to increase the circulation, mobility, and flexibility of the tendon and modify the tension of the muscles.

ACHILLES TENDON

Work locally along the course of the Achilles tendon. Ask where the patient feels the most pain and work more intensely on the painful area, usually the mid-portion of the tendon. You might also need to work on the whole leg, especially on the gastrocnemius and soleus.

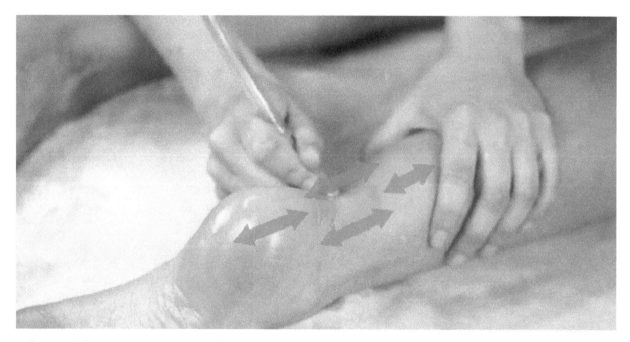

Image 19-1: Main treatment areas when treating the Achilles tendon. Work on all sides of the tendon and you might also need to treat the whole leg, especially the gastrocnemius and soleus.

QUADRICEPS TENDON

Problems with this tendon are more common in athletes in sports that require jumping, deep lunges, running, and quick stop and starts. It is also called "Patellofemoral Pain Syndrome," and in adolescents *Sinding Larsen Syndrome*. Not to be compared to Osgood-Schlatter disease, which is an inflammatory disease of the insertion of the quadriceps tendon on the tibial tuberosity.

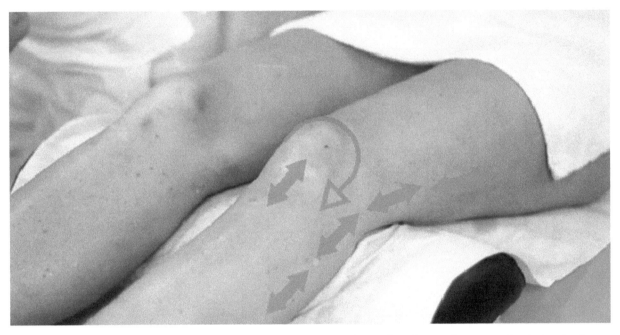

Image 19-2: Treatment areas for "jumper's" and "runner's" knee when the quadriceps tendon is involved.

ADDUCTOR TENDONS

The adductor muscles are composed of the adductor magnus, brevis, minimus, and longus, in addition to gracilis, pectineus. Problems with this tendon are often common after or during pregnancy, kicking sports, and with ice skaters, for example. The pain is usually located in the groin. Work directly on the tendons, but also the psoas and adductor muscle belly.

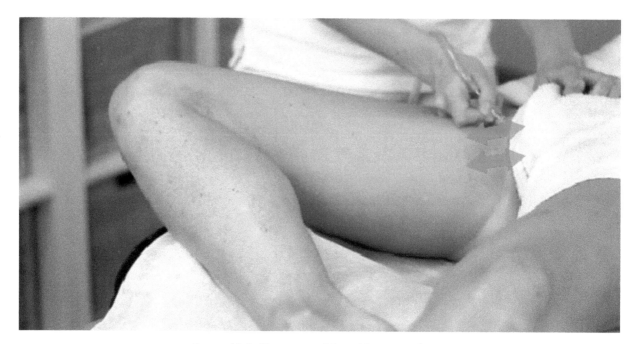

Image 19-3: Treatment of the adductor tendon.

TENDON OF FOREARM

Humans have approximately 20 tendons in the forearm, depending on how the anatomy is interpreted in terms of the function of the tendons. Here we will only mention the tendons most commonly affected.

One of the most common tendinopathies is called "Tennis Elbow," which is an irritation of the extensor carpi radialis brevis. Curiously, the insertion of this tendon is about 50 percent in diameter compared to extensor carpi radialis longus. And they are considered to be able to generate the same amount of force, hence most tendinopathies are located in the extensor radialis brevis.

"Golfer's Elbow" is basically the same problem, but less common, and located on the medial side of the elbow. It involves the common flexor origin where the pronator teres, flexor carpi radialis, flexor carpi ulnaris, flexor digitorum superficialis, and palmaris longus inserts on the medial epicondyle of the humerus.

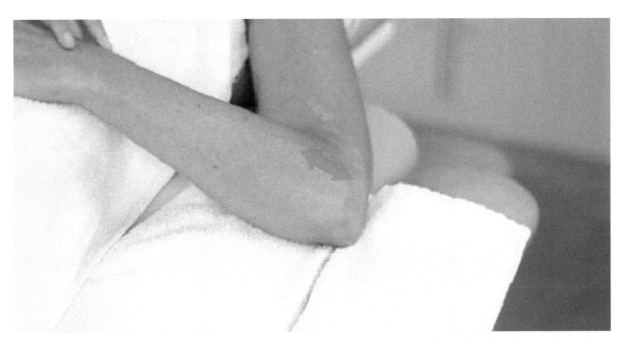

Image 19-4: Treatment of the Extensor Carpi Radialis Brevis tendon (tennis elbow). Work on the tendon and insertion, but it is usually beneficial to include the muscles in the forearm and sometimes also the upper arm.

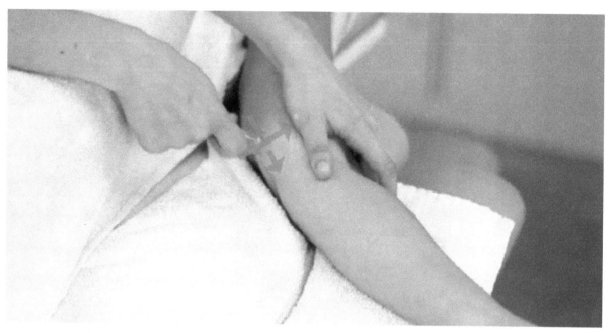

Image 19-5: Treatment of the Common Flexor origin (Golfer's Elbow). Work on the tendons, but also all the muscles in forearm and sometimes also the upper arm.

[20] NERVES AND NERVE ENTRAPMENT

The nervous system is a complex and awe-inspiring system that we are probably far away from gaining a full understanding of, but we will provide a brief explanation here. The nervous system is the signaling system of the body. It can almost be compared to an electrical system—an electric cord, supplying electricity to an electric device. It is divided into the central nervous system (brain and spinal cord), and the peripheral nervous system (peripheral nerves). Nerves are divided into motor (efferent) and sensory (afferent). Some nerves are purely motor, some sensory, and others are capable of both.

We will not focus on systemic diseases that can affect the function of the nervous system like Multiple Sclerosis (MS) or Amyotrophic Lateral Sclerosis (ALS).

Nerve injuries are commonly due to compression of the nerve itself. For example, a spinal disc herniation may compress the nerve root, causing pain and/or change in motor and sensory signaling, along the affected nerve distribution. Depending on the level of the compression, different symptoms are usually displayed. In general, we divide this into three categories:

1. Central compression (spinal disc herniation, lateral recess stenosis) leads to pain (primary symptom), numbness (secondary symptom), "pins and needles" (tertiary symptom).

2. Plexus compression (bracial plexus, for example) leads to pins and needles, pain, numbness.

3. Distal nerve compression (carpal tunnel syndrome, for example) leads to numbness, pins and needles, pain.

CENTRAL COMPRESSION

The most common affected areas are the cervical nerves of C7, and to a lesser extent C6. In the lumbar region S1 is most commonly affected. L5 is common. L4 less common, and L3 rare. Note that spinal disc herniation in the thoracic region is rare.

The symptoms correspond to the level of the nerve. So compression of the C7 nerve-root can cause pain, numbness and pins and needles in the corresponding dermatome. Also, muscles supplied by the C7 nerve-root may be weaker. Usually for the C7 nerve-root this is loss of power in the triceps and flexors of the wrist.

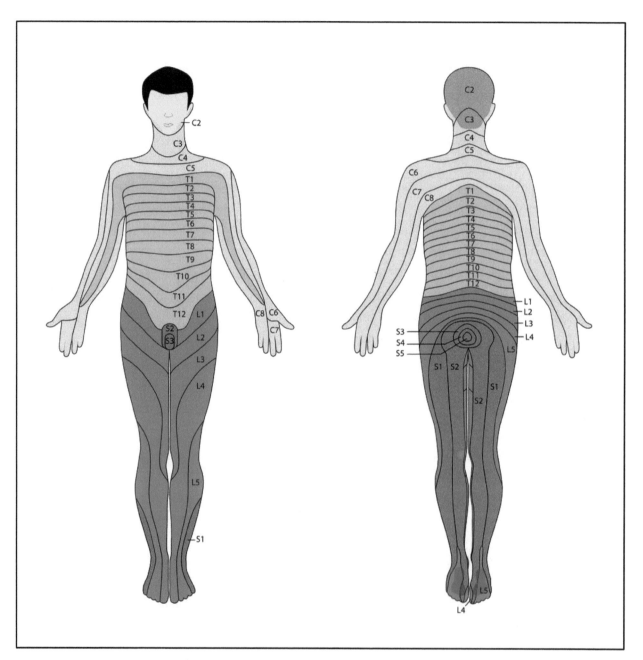

Image 20-1: Dermatomes corresponding to nerve-root levels.

TREATMENT

If the cause of the compression is a spinal disc herniation, this cannot be altered using the Tuxen Method. However, treatment is aimed at modifying symptoms. Work on the corresponding spinal level in the neck or the lower back. Try to follow the nerve course, and work on muscles that the nerve runs along or through.

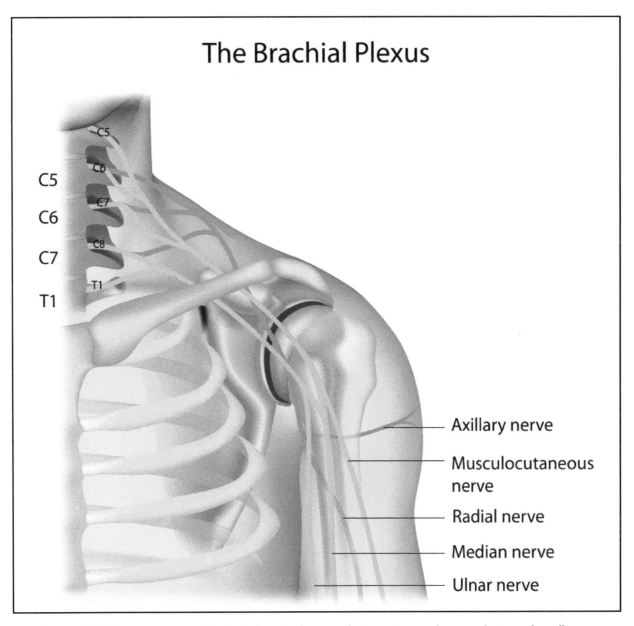

Image 20-2: The most commonly affected cervical nerves that can give numbness and pins and needles.

PLEXUS

Thoracic outlet syndrome (TOS) is the most commonly affected plexus problem. Most patients have what is called a symptomatic TOS, where they have the symptoms of numbness and/or pins and needles, but MRI and x-rays are usually negative. True TOS is a structural change, for example an extra rib that is compressing the nerve, and this is very unusual. Symptomatic TOS is usually caused by tight or over-active pectoralis minor or scalene muscles. Posture may also be a cause, and should not be missed. People with symptomatic TOS usually respond well to the Tuxen Method treatment.

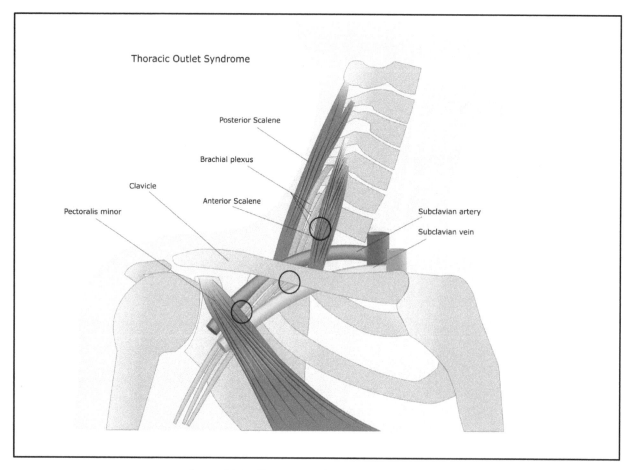

Image 20-3: Thoracic Outlet Syndrome (TOS).

TREATMENT (TOS)

Treat the scalene and pectoralis minor. Also include the trapezius, levator scapulae, rhomboid and pectoralis major. If posture is a contributing factor in the patient's TOS, include muscles that are identified as barriers to a good posture.

CARPAL TUNNEL SYNDROME (MEDIAN NERVE)

This a local entrapment of the nerves in the carpal tunnel of the wrist. Risk factors are obesity, repetitive wrist work, risks to pregnancy, and rheumatoid arthritis. Symptoms are often numbness and pain in the first three fingers, and the radial half of the fourth finger. If you tap on the wrist over the carpal tunnel (called the "Tinel test"), this may reproduce symptoms.

TREATMENT

Work over the carpal tunnel and include the general palmar area. Work from distal to centrally.

ATHLETES

[21] TUXEN METHOD FOR ATHLETES

THE SPORTS ATHLETE

In this chapter we will show how you can help athletes and other active clients by treating and preventing sports injuries. We also demonstrate how to optimize recovery after training.

Sport medicine is a vast area of knowledge, so it is far beyond the scope of this book to cover even a small portion. However, we want to focus on how treatment with the Tuxen Method may be used as a clinical tool primarily on muscle and joint injuries.

Athletes range from the elite to the weekend performer. In general we divide between preventable and unpreventable injuries. Injuries that can be prevented are usually related to overuse and overtraining, while various sports have inherent risks associated with them. Consider an American football player that is tackled at knee-height, and sustains a partial rupture to their medial collateral ligament. This is an injury that cannot be prevented, at least not as a musculo-skeletal therapist. Hence, our role is to prevent small injuries from increasing in severity through early intervention, and speed up the healing process when an athlete experiences an acute injury.

Anamnesis and examinations should reveal which structure is a fault. This is sometimes no simple task, but one can use experience and clinical reasoning to find the correct area.

Acute injury often requires PRICE-principle application , especially with severe swelling.

These principles are usually applied from 0-48 hours immediately after the injury. The goal is to reduce swelling, prevent further injury, and reduce pain.

- Protection

- Rest

- Ice

- Compression

- Elevation

GENERAL ADVICE ON TRAUMA

Traumatic injuries are frequent in some sports with high speed, in contact sports, and those with demanding movements.

In general, sudden pain, a high degree of swelling, and an inability to weight-bear, may indicate fracture and/or ligamentous injury. Unless you work in a sports setting, these patients may be rare in you practice. But keep in mind that fractures may be overlooked. Small fractures are not always that simple to diagnose, especially stress fractures. Carefully consider the patient's history and the expected rate of recovery. For example, small fractures of the lower limb tend not to heal as quickly as a sprained ankle. Refer to a medical doctor if in doubt.

Also, symptoms of pins and needles, tingling or numbness after acute injury, or partial or full loss of strength, should be referred to a medical doctor, as this may result from an injured nerve or partial/full rupture of a muscle or tendon.

FEAR AVOIDANCE AND COMPENSATORY MECHANISMS

Athletes need to trust that their bodies can withstand the load while performing. If an injury occurs that the athlete struggles to overcome, this may alter the kinetic chain to decrease use of the injured or previously injured area. Consequently, this may lead to overuse of another area or to a decrease in performance.

For example an athlete with longstanding lower back pain may tend toward increased use of the hip or knee joint, thereby loading these joints and surrounding muscles more. Another example would be a baseball pitcher with pain in the thoracic spine during rotation. In order to generate the same amount of force, torque must be produced somewhere else in the kinetic chain. For a pitcher this is usually the shoulder, which in turn increases the load on the shoulder joint. In general, the more symmetrical the athlete in muscle length and strength, the less risk of injury.

Always assess the flexibility of an athlete after injury, especially after prolonged issues. Also, try to ascertain if the athlete has developed any compensatory mechanisms.

WHEN A MASSAGE THERAPIST CAN HELP WITH ACUTE PAIN

(See chapter 6 about pain.)

- Acute pain without injury

- Acute pain without swelling in joint or muscle

- Acute pain without severe loss of muscle force

- Acute pain without numbness or tingling

Other conditions may also be beneficial for the massage therapist to treat, but you want to have had other specialists look upon the patient also.

GENERAL PRINCIPLES FOR ACUTE INJURIES

If the athlete has a severe swelling, use principles of drainage.

Assess which movement is painful or problematic, treat one area, and reassess the movement to ensure the correct areas have been targeted.

Use the following principles:

1. Decrease swelling

2. Increase circulation

3. Increase flexibility

Start gently and gradually increase intensity if tolerable. Work around the injured area initially. Apply gentle trigger-point treatment with the vacuum cup on the most painful area. A smaller cup may be used depending on the severity of the injury. Ice may be used after treatment to prevent increase of swelling for 5-10 minutes.

Vacuum therapy requires less time than massage for one area to be stimulated sufficiently to generate a therapeutic effect, so don't over treat.

ACUTE LOWER BACK PAIN

Consider history. For example, a hard football tackle, a fall, or a high-velocity injury may cause a fracture. If in doubt, consult a medical doctor.

Commonly, patients will present bi- or unilateral pain with pain on forward and/or side-bending.

Although acute lower-back pain may originate from the lumbar disc or the facet joint, treating the muscles may result in considerable improvement as these muscles tend to reflectively co-contract.

As long as the pain does not radiate below the knee you may decrease the athlete's pain significantly during the first session.

1. Identify muscles contributing to patient's complaint by assessing movement, muscle tone and tenderness on palpation.

2. Primary muscles: erector spina, psoas, iliacus, quadratus lumborum.

3. Secondary muscles: gluteus maximus and medius, latissimus dorsi, thoracic part of erector spina, transversus abdominus, diaphragm, hamstring.

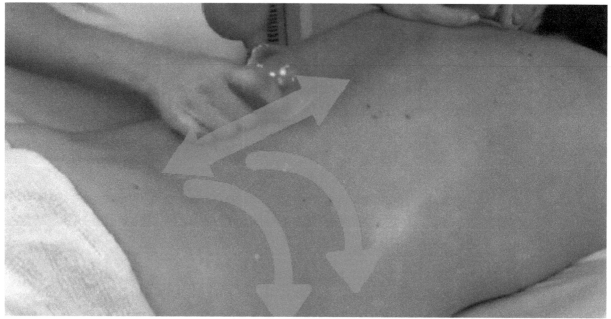

Image 21-1: Picture demonstrating treatment of the primary muscles: erector spina, psoas, iliacus and the quadratus lumborum.

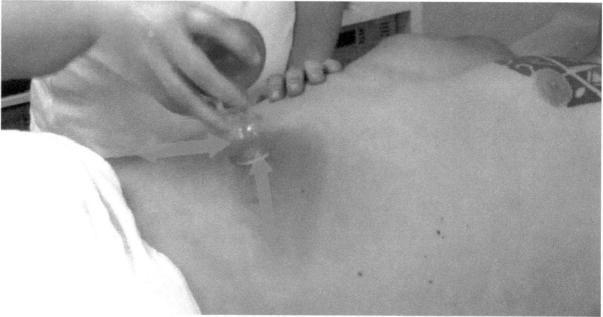

Image 21-2: Figure showing indirect treatment of psoas via the abdominal area from umbilicus to the superior anterior iliac crest.

CHRONIC LOWER BACK PAIN

Chronic lower back pain is now considered as a more bio-psycho-social aspect, but here we focus on how to apply the Tuxen Method. We apply the same principles as with acute lower back pain, but the athlete may need additional treatments to fully recover.

The effect of the treatment is cumulative, so typically 3-5 sessions with a week's rest between treatments (time for the bruise to heal) is recommended.

1. Identify muscles contributing to patient's complaint by assessing movement, muscle tone and tenderness on palpation.

2. Primary muscles: erector spina, psoas, iliacus, quadratus lumborum.

3. Secondary muscles: gluteus maximus and medius, latissimus dorsi, thoracic part of erector spina, transversus abdominius, diaphragm, hamstring.

THORACIC PAIN

The thoracic spine is an important force transmitter and generator in sports, so assessment of thoracic flexibility of the area is important.

Often patients have pain on rotation, inhaling and/or exhaling.

Beware of fractured ribs. Consult a medical doctor if in doubt.

1. Identify muscles contributing to patient's complaint by assessing movement, muscle tone and tenderness on palpation.

2. Primary muscles: thoracic part of erector spina, rhomboid, lower trapezius, middle trapezius, intercostal muscles.

3. Secondary muscles: diaphragm, pectoralis minor, serratus anterior, upper trapezius, lumbar and cervical part of erector spina.

SHORTNESS OF BREATH IN ATHLETES

A sensation of insufficient inhalation during exercise may be due to tight or over-active diaphragm, intercostals, and rigid thoracic spine

Vacuum therapy can be helpful in increasing the respiratory function.

Numerous diseases may affect the respiratory function, so consider referring to a medical doctor.

1. Identify muscles contributing to patient's complaint by assessing movement, muscle tone and tenderness on palpation.

2. Primary muscles: thoracic part of erector spina, intercostal muscles, diaphragm.

3. Secondary muscles: pectoralis minor, serratus anterior, trapezius, lumbar and cervical part of erector spina.

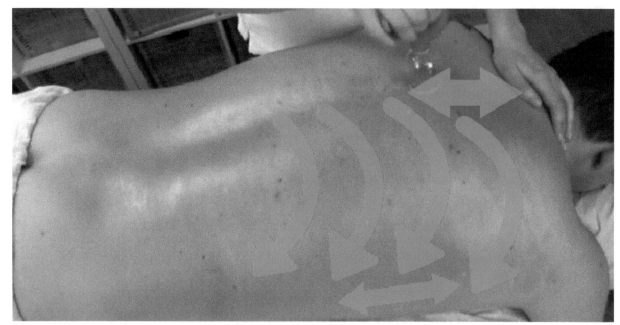

Image 21-3: Figure showing treatment of the primary back muscles needing treatment when there is thoracic pain or shortness of breath.

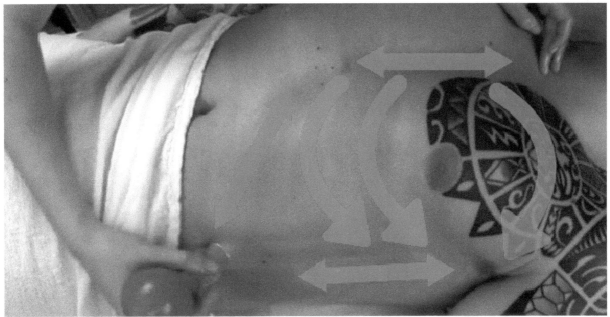

Image 21-4: Figure showing treatment of the primary frontal muscles for thoracic pain or shortness of breath.

ACUTE HAMSTRING PAIN

Usually acute pain and loss of function related to sport at the proximal part or the middle of the semimembranosus.

Swelling is not uncommon, and is indicative of a tear. Vacuum therapy will often help, but athlete will need rehabilitation to rebuild strength and to prevent future injuries.

With tears you may feel the compromised area where the actual tear has occurred with palpation. A full tear is rare, but lack of ability to weight-bear, significantly reduced strength, swelling with discoloring, are the clinical signs of a full rupture.

1. Identify muscles contributing to patient's complaint by assessing movement, muscle tone and tenderness on palpation.

2. Primary muscles: hamstring (usually semimembranosus).

3. Secondary muscles: gluteus maximus and medius, piriformis, obturator internus/externus, popliteus, gastrocnemius.

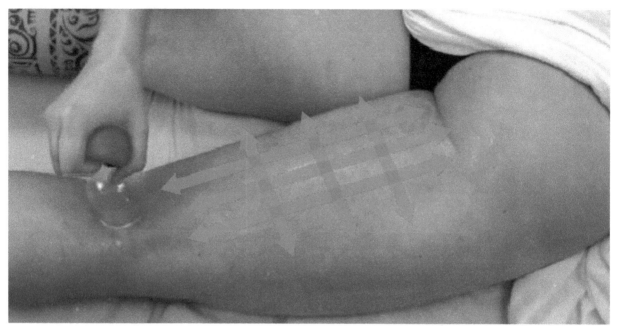

Image 21-5: Figure showing treatment of the hamstring.

LEG PAIN

Injuries in the leg are usually located dorsally, medially, or antero-medially.

Dorsally: usually the gastrocnemius, but the plantaris or soleus may also be at fault.

1. Identify muscles contributing to patient's complaint by assessing movement, muscle tone and tenderness on palpation.

2. Primary muscles: gastrocnemius (usually the medial head), plantaris, soleus.

3. Secondary muscles: hamstring, gluteus maximus.

Note: If the patient displays symptoms like swelling, warmth and/or redness without trauma, be aware of Deep Venous Thrombosis. Immediate medical attention is required.

Laterally: overuse of the peroneal muscles. Note that these are part of the lateral compartment in the leg. Longstanding problems that do not improve with conservative treatment may need a surgical fascial release.

1. Identify muscles contributing to patient's complaint by assessing movement, muscle tone and tenderness on palpation.

2. Primary muscles: peroneus brevis and longus.

3. Secondary muscles: tensor fascia lata, quadriceps, gastrocnemius, lateral part gluteus maximus and gluteus medius.

Antero-medial:

Tibialis anterior is a common source of leg pain. This is considered an overuse injury, and is usually related to running. Consider footwear and total milage. The tibialis anterior is part of the anterior compartment of the leg. Longstanding problems that do not improve with conservative treatment may need a surgical fascial release.

1. Identify muscles contributing to patient's complaint by assessing movement, muscle tone and tenderness on palpation.

2. Primary muscles: tibialis anterior.

3. Secondary muscles: extensor digitorum longus, extensor hallucis longus, peroneus tertius, quadriceps.

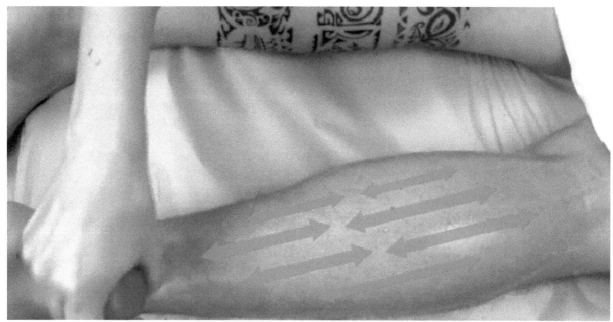

Image 21-6: Figure showing primary treatment area in leg pain.

HIP PAIN IN ATHLETES

Note that joint problems are quite common for athletes in the hip. Examples are labral tears, stress fractures, osteoarthritis and FAI (Femoral Acetabular Impingement. These conditions cannot be cured with the Tuxen Method, but symptoms may be modified. However, consider referring to a medical doctor. Also refer to a medical doctor if you suspect a Slipped Capital Femoral Epiphysis (SCFE) or Perthes disease in a young patient.

Muscle injuries are common in the hip. These are usually overuse related, and may require rehabilitation for strengthening and prevention of future injuries. Acute injuries is usually located anteriorly or medially.

Anterior:

1. Identify muscles contributing to patient's complaint by assessing movement, muscle tone and tenderness on palpation.

2. Primary muscles: psoas, iliacus.

3. Secondary muscles: quadriceps, sartorius, rectus abdominis, internal/external oblique.

Medially:

1. Identify muscles contributing to patient's complaint by assessing movement, muscle tone and tenderness on palpation.

2. Primary muscles: adductor longus, adductor brevis, adductor magnus, pectineus, gracilis.

3. Secondary muscles: quadriceps, piriformis, gemelli muscles.

Lateral:

1. Identify muscles contributing to patient's complaint by assessing movement, muscle tone and tenderness on palpation.

2. Primary muscles: gluteus medius, tensor fascia lata, lateral part gluteus maximus.

3. Secondary muscles: quadratus lumborum, gluteus maximus, psoas, iliacus, quadriceps.

Posterior:

1. Identify muscles contributing to patient's complaint by assessing movement, muscle tone and tenderness on palpation.

2. Primary muscles: Gluteus maximus, quadratus femoris, piriformis,

3. Secondary muscles: Lumbar part erector spina, hamstring, latissimus dorsi, quadratus lumborum.

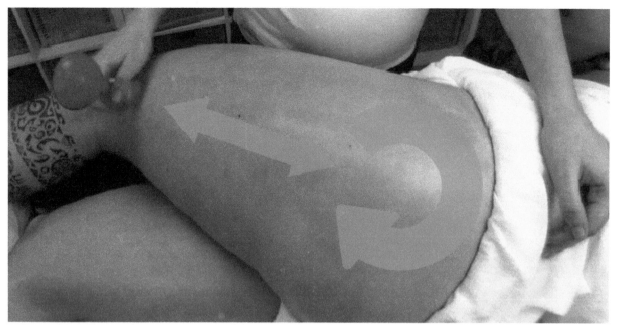

Image 21-7: Figure showing treatment of the primary muscles: gluteus medius, tensor fascia lata, lateral part gluteus maximus.

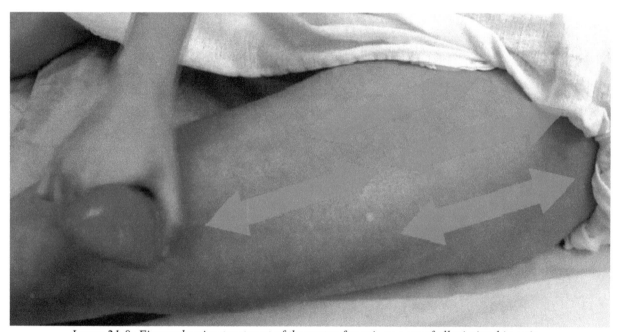

Image 21-8: Figure showing treatment of the rectus femoris as part of alleviating hip pain.

SHOULDER PAIN

Shoulder pain is one of the most common sites for injuries of athletes. Note that joint problems in the shoulder are quite common for athletes. Examples are dislocations, labral tears, and fractures. Consider referring to a medical doctor if you suspect a significant joint injury. Shoulder injuries commonly need rehabilitation to strengthen and prevent future injury.

Anterior:

1. Identify muscles contributing to patient's complaint by assessing movement, muscle tone and muscle pain on palpation.

2. Primary muscles: subscapularis, biceps.

3. Secondary muscles: pectoralis minor, pectoralis major, deltoid, subclavius, lower trapezius, serratus anterior.

Lateral:

1. Identify muscles contributing to patient's complaint by assessing movement, muscle tone and muscle pain on palpation.

2. Primary muscles: supraspinatus, infraspinatus.

3. Secondary muscles: upper trapezius, rhomboid, serratus anterior, teres minor and major, latissimus dorsi, pectoralis minor and major.

Posterior:

1. Identify muscles contributing to patient's complaint by assessing movement, muscle tone and muscle pain on palpation.

2. Primary muscles: infraspinatus, rhomboid, teres minor.

3. Secondary muscles: teres major, latissimus dorsi, trapezius, pectoralis minor and major, levator scapula.

ACUTE SWELLING OF A JOINT

Acute swelling requires PRICE-principle application. Beware of fractures or ligamentous injury. Consult a medical doctor if in doubt. Signs of fracture include significant swelling, significant and sudden pain, and inability to weight-bear.

Vacuum therapy is an effective method to decrease swelling. The severity of the injury dictates when vacuum therapy is best applied. With a small injury, meaning slight swelling and low/medium pain, you can start treatment the same day. But in more severe cases, it may be better to wait between 24-72 hours. Use your clinical judgment and communicate well with your patient.

Always work distally to proximally. Start working around the injured area, and gradually work towards the central part of the swelling. When treating directly over the injured area, start with a small cup with low intensity. Gradually work deeper into the swelling.

Consider applying cold cream or similar products for pain control, and ice or compression after treatment. This usually requires 1-5 sessions depending on severity. The most common joints to receive injury are the ankle and the knee.

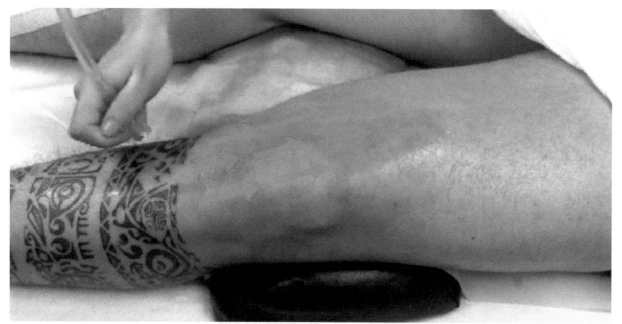

Image 21-9: Picture demonstrating vacuum therapy to decrease swelling. Always work distally to proximally.

THE INFLEXIBLE ATHLETE

Flexibility varies from individual to individual and is the result of genetic predisposition and use of the body. Some sports require a large degree of movement in some joints, others do not. In some sports it is beneficial to have flexibility of certain joints. Consider a baseball pitcher's external rotation of the shoulder. Whereas in contrast, for a weight lifter it is not beneficial to have a high degree of flexibility on their shoulders as they need to provide sufficient stability.

If an athlete needs more flexibility in an area of their body, vacuum therapy may help. Restriction or decreased flexibility often arise after an injury. By working on fascia and muscles this may increase. Keep in mind that often a decreased range of movement is the inability to decrease tone of the antagonists of the respective movement. For example, forward bending requires the hamstring to decrease in activity. By treating the hamstring, you often quite dramatically increase the range of forward bending. Apply this principle when helping the inflexible athlete. Consider which movements and muscles need correction.

RECOVERY

Recovery is vital to the elite athlete. Prolonged recovery results in less training hours and perhaps a decrease in training quality.

General benefits for applying recovery vacuum therapy:

- May aid in soft tissue recovery.

- Decrease of DOMS (delayed onset muscle soreness after exercise).

- Vacuum therapy may increase circulation to damaged tissue.

- High training load may result in increased muscle tone in rest and during movement. Vacuum therapy may help normalize the muscle tone after exercise.

- Increased muscle tone also decreases the shock absorbency capacity of the soft tissue, resulting in increased risk of injury.

- Abnormal high tone has been hypothesized to impair the delivery of nutrition and oxygen and hamper the removal of metabolites.

- May also reverse biomechanical abnormalities, especially if this is asymmetrical.

- Increased muscle tone may also elicit fatigue in muscle and increasing the recovery time.

RECOVERY MASSAGE TECHNIQUE 1

This technique should be used shortly before competition or in between each competition, matches or competing days. This is often used in a tournament or competition with little time between each event.

Apply a low dosage and do not create severe bruising, as high-dosage vacuum therapy may cause soreness which may affect the athlete's performance.

It is beneficial if you work with the same athlete over time, as you learn the tissue-response of that particular person. It is advised to stay below 4 on the VAS-score.

Cold water immersion (ice bath) or deep water running after treatment may aid in recovery.

RECOVERY VACUUM TECHNIQUE 2

This technique should be applied in lower-load exercise periods.

Use higher dosage vacuum therapy throughout the whole body and focus on problem areas, especially areas where the athlete has a history of injury. This often creates bruising, but in a low-load period of training, the body can easily cope with the added short-term load.

Athlete can exercise the same day as a treatment, but the athlete may experience more tiredness or soreness after a training-session.

BENEFITS OF TECHNIQUE 2 FOR RECOVERY

- Bruising may increase the capillaries' capability to transport blood more effectively, making the athlete less prone to muscle soreness over time.

- Deep vacuum therapy may increase the flexibility of the muscles to aid in movement optimization.

- One area should not be stimulated before bruising has vanished. This usually occurs between 2-10 days.

- When re-treating an area, the area usually recovers more quickly as less restructuring of the capillary system is required.

- Remember to co-operate with the athlete and coaching-team to ensure the timing of treatments fit with the scheduled training plan.

Failing to plan is planning to fail!

THE FATIGUED ATHLETE/OVERTRAINING SYNDROME

Often athletes total load over time surpasses the body's ability to cope with the stresses. This is a complicated process, not only encompassing the physical aspect, but also the psychological and social aspect. Many of the world's top athletes have an entire team of professionals surrounding them to aid in these matters.

Signs and symptoms:

- General feeling of tiredness and excessive fatigue when exercising.

- "Too much too much, too soon and too often."

- Increased lactic acid buildup during training.

- Subjective feeling of heaviness when exercising.

- Prolonged recovery periods after competition or training and increased DOMS.

- Inability to reach maximal heart rate, and higher heart rate in rest.

- Decreased motivation or sleep disturbance.

Athlete should consult a medical doctor to check nutrition levels and general health. Consult nutritionist if required. Ask the athlete to consult their trainer to review exercise load.

HOW TO HELP THE FATIGUED ATHLETE

Vacuum therapy increases the blood flow to the capillaries and therefore the muscles. It also increases the ability to get rid of metabolics/lactic acid after exercising. Re-building the capillary system can increase recovery and performance, thereby increasing the athlete's confidence in his body. This can be an important first step towards peak performance.

- Consider treating the whole body, especially the area where the symptoms are felt (e.g. tiredness in legs or thighs during running).

- Usually needs at least 10 treatments on the most affected areas for full recovery.

- Start gently with low dosage, and gradually increase.

- Tight muscles and decreased blood flow throughout the whole legs.

- The athlete may need some rest from exercise after deep vacuum therapy due to longer recovery period than normal.

- It is important that the other factors mentioned are addressed to ensure optimal results.

[22] THERAPY FOR SPECIFIC ATHLETES

THE BIKER

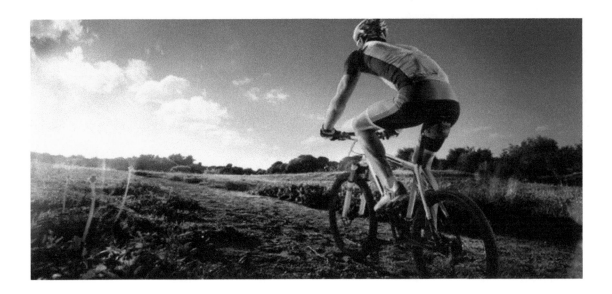

Often tight or overactive:

- Pectoral

- Cervical extensors

- Hamstring

- Psoas

- Tibialis anterior

Tight frontal sling due to repetitive flexion in the hip and trunk and posterior sling due to prolonged flexion in the knee and cervical posture on the bike. A professional adjustment of the bike is advised if biking a substantial number of hours during a week.

THE SWIMMER

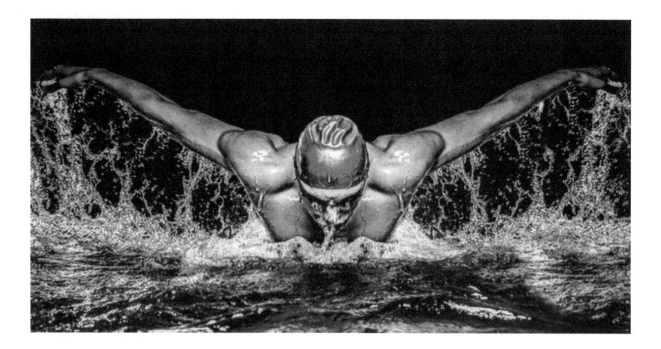

In general, swimmers don't usually have issues with joint mobility, probably due to the fact that they repeat the same motion over and over again, enabling the tissue to adapt. In contrast, they are more prone to multidirectional instability of the shoulder. Hence more commonly, they suffer from overuse injuries, especially in the shoulder.

Common problems include:

- Overuse supraspinatus and biceps longus.

- Muscle imbalance internal rotators and adductors shoulder vs. external rotators and scapular stabilizers.

- Lower back problems, especially breast and butterfly-swimmers.

- Medial collateral ligament stress syndrome- breast strokers.

THE GOLFER

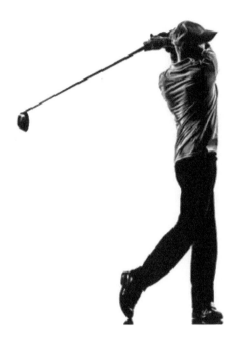

Golf, depending on the level, requires a high-speed recoil of the entire body. Assess where the limiting factor may lie, and treat this region first. Professional coaching is important.

Common problems:

- Lower back pain, especially in the last phase of the swing

- Inadequate rotation in e.g. hips, will require other parts of the body to rotate more and potentially causing problems

- Shoulders

- Knees

- Decreased rotation of the thoracic spine

THE HORSEBACK RIDER

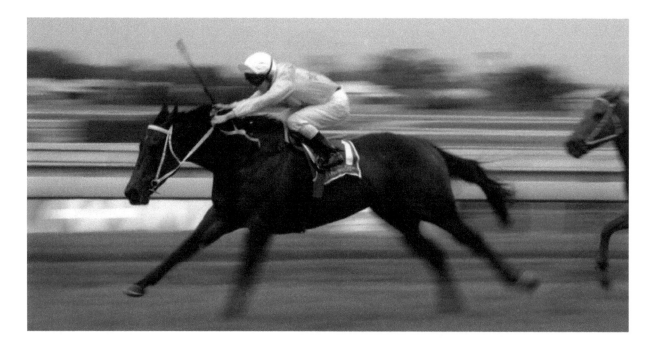

Riding puts a lot of strain on the hip muscles, especially the adductors. The term "riders sprain" indicates overuse of the adductor muscles.

Common problems:

- Adductor muscles

- Hip rotators (which generate stability, especially the external rotators)

- Pectoralis major

- Abdominal muscles

- Infraspinatus/teres minor

- Lower back muscles

THE GYMNAST AND THE DANCER

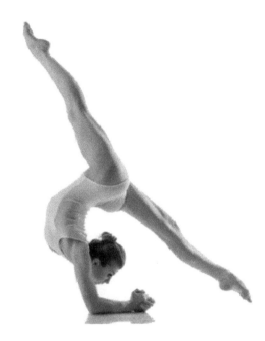

These are perhaps two of the most challenging sports for the human body. They require strength, endurance, balance, control, and flexibility. Some gymnasts and dancers are highly specialized, so consider which movements the patient does on a regular basis. Confer with a trainer to find faulty movement patterns that may have developed. Attempt to restore function by addressing the limiting factors.

Common problems:

- Acute injuries

- Overuse, especially shoulders and knees

- Lower back

THE RUNNER

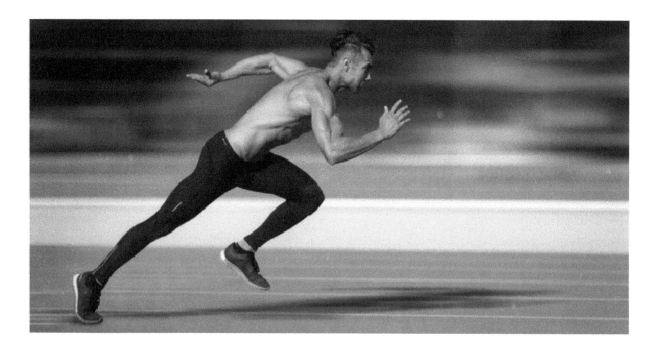

Runners are prone to overuse of the lower extremity. Non-professionals often progress too rapidly with their total mileage per week with insufficient rest. The typical running patient is a 40-year-old male that has recently started running or returned to running after a long hiatus. Consider referring to a running coach.

Common problems:

- Hip problems (gluteus medius, psoas and adductors)

- Knee (runner's knee, jumper's knee)

- Achilles tendinopathy

- Lower back pain

THE TENNIS PLAYER

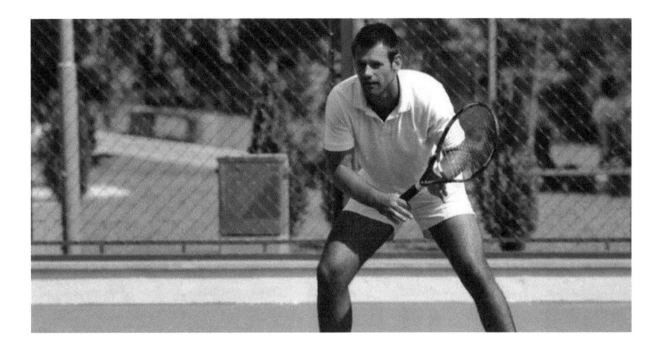

Tennis is a demanding sport at high levels. For amateurs, the largest stress is usually on the shoulder joint, especially during the serve. Confer with a tennis trainer, and try to assess which movement is associated with the patient's problem.

Common problems:

- Shoulder pain. Instability vs. overuse. The more flexibility the joint has, the more stability the rotator cuff has to provide.

- Overuse achilles, hip muscles and lower back.

- Inadequate rotation of hips and trunk requiring more force to be transmitted through the shoulder joint.

[23] TREATING THE MOST COMMON SPORTS INJURIES

RUNNER'S KNEE

"Runner's knee" is a pain in the lateral side of knee, usually where the iliotibial band glides over the lateral condyle of the femur. Some consider this an overuse injury, while others have a more biomechanical interpretation often referring to a tight or short iliotibial band and running technique. It is common in cyclists and runners.

Treatment: Release the iliotibial band, gluteus medius, tensor fascia lata, lateral part of gluteus maximus.

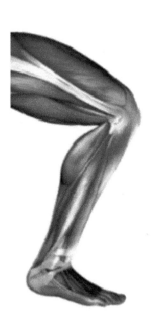 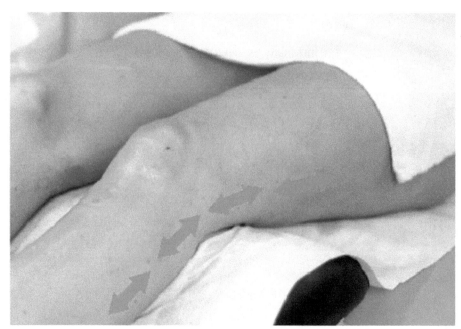

Image 23-1: The ITB band and the area to work on.

PATELLOFEMORAL PAIN SYNDROME (PFPS)

Frequent injury in jumping sports, sprinting, or fast running (such as football, etc.), PFPS is an overload of the quadriceps tendon where it encompasses the patella, usually in the distal region.

Treatment: Release the tendon, quadriceps, pectineus, psoas and hamstring.

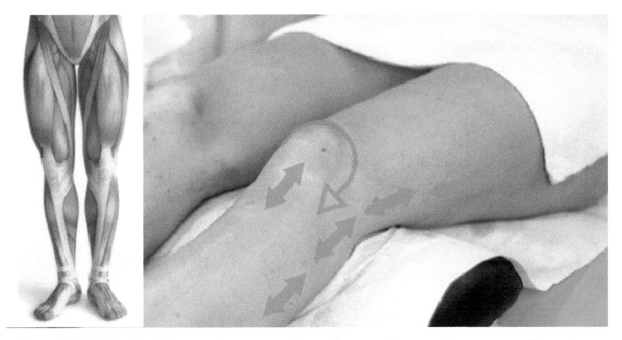

Image 23-2: ITB band and the area where to treat. Also work on quadriceps, pectineus, psoas and hamstring.

TENNIS LEG

"Tennis Leg" is a sudden onset of pain in the middle part of the calf. This is usually due to a partial rupture of the plantaris or medial head of the gastrocnemius. Apply PRICE-principle (Protection-Rest-Ice-Compression-Elevation) for acute treatment.

Treat the gastrocnemius, plantaris and soleus.

Note: Tennis leg may mimic Deep Venous Thrombosis (DVT), but be aware that DVT requires immediate medical attention.

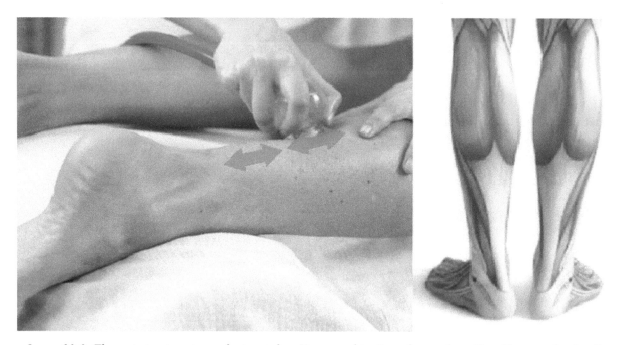

Image 23-3: The main treatment area for tennis leg. Use a combination of several small and long strokes in all directions. You can also use a static technique with higher pressure at the site of the lesion.

GENERAL TEARS

Partial tears in a muscle often cause sudden and sharp pain and are a relatively common injury in sports—in particular, sports with high speed and acceleration. The tear is usually in the musculo-tendinous area of the muscles or the muscle belly itself. There might be signs of bleeding and/or bruises of muscle fibers which have ruptured.

TREATING PARTIAL TEARS WITH THE TUXEN METHOD

If in the acute stage, start with mild strokes over the whole muscle to decrease the tension and help drain away the fluid. After 2-3 weeks you can apply more aggressive treatment to promote circulation and healing. Often 2-3 treatments is enough to see improvement. Start superficially and then go deeper with a larger vacuum cup. Consider prescribing gentle exercises to gradually load the area.

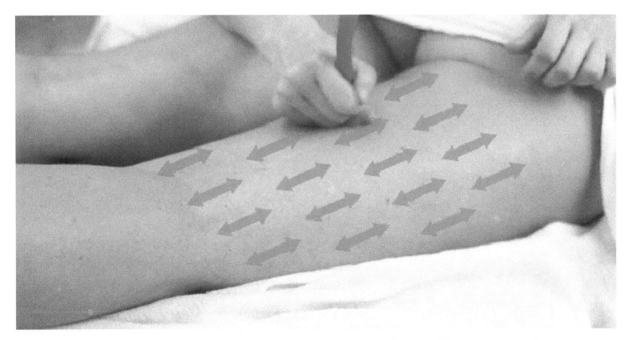

Image 23-4: Scanning the leg to locate the tear. The injured area will bruise more easily.

SHIN SPLINTS

Shin splints are often the result of overuse, of either the tibialis anterior or posterior muscle. If the tibialis anterior is the symptomatic structure, pain will be located on the lateral side of the tibia, while tibialis posterior will cause pain on the medial part of the tibia.

Shin splints are often caused by overuse related to running, as the tibialis anterior provides the eccentric force during landing of the foot, while the tibialis posterior provide stability during landing. If you suspect the running technique of the patient may be a cause of the problem, refer to a running coach. Also, pay attention to the running shoes used. Consider referring to a competent salesperson of running shoes.

Treatment: Tibialis anterior and posterior. Consider ventral and lateral fascial sling.

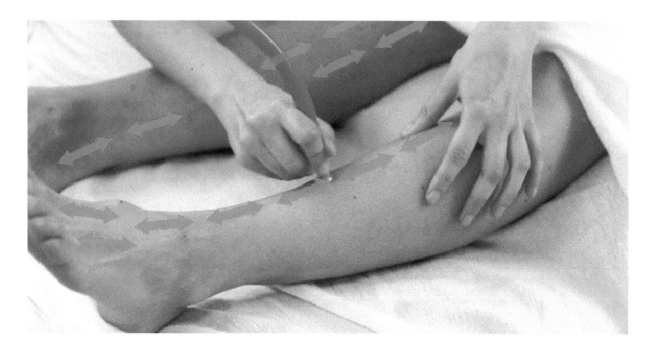

Image 23-5: Treatment of tibialis anterior and posterior.

GOLFERS AND TENNIS ELBOWS

Golfer's Elbow (common flexor origin) and Tennis Elbow (extensor carpi radialis brevis) are names for the two most common tendinopathies in the lower arm. Pain is usually caused by resisted wrist movements. Sometimes overuse of the respective muscles elicit pain below the insertion.

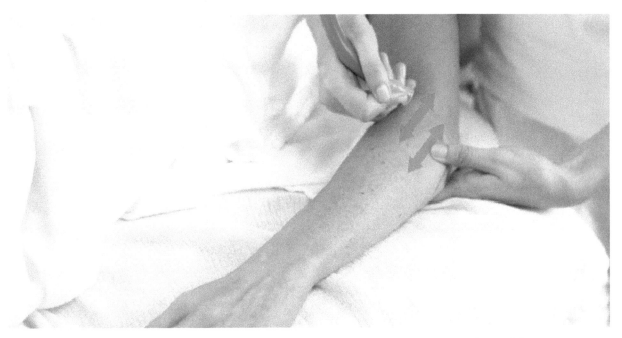

Image 23-6: Treatment area for Tennis Elbow. Also treat the muscle if pain is located there.

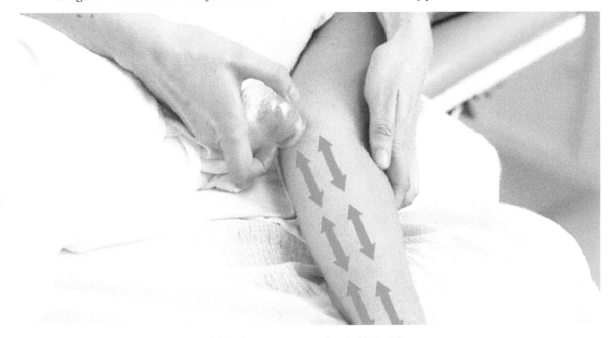

Image 23-7: Treatment area for Golfer's Elbow.

AREAS & ASPECTS

[24] CERVICAL AND TENSION HEADACHE

TENSION HEADACHE

Tension headache may be attributed to muscle tension around the neck, jaw, or head. Some research suggest that changes in processing of pain signals may be a contributing cause. Tension headache usually feels like a tight band around the head. The tension is mostly bilateral and circular. Although tension headache has been associated with different disorders, such as a cluster headache or migraine, these may coexist. The most common muscles that can contribute to tension headache are:

From neck:

- Trapezius

- Levator scapula

- Rhomboid minor and major

- Extensor muscles of the upper cervical spine (semispinalis capitis, iliocostalis cervicis, longissimus cervicis, longissimus capitis)

Muscles around head:

- Jaw (temporalis, masseter)

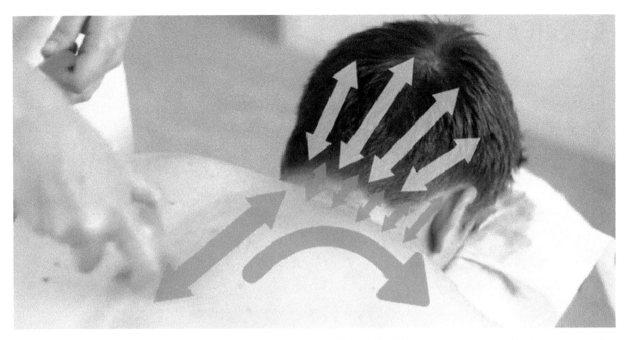

Image 24-1: Treatment areas posteriorly for treating tension headache. To treat areas covered by hair, you need a vacuum machine to generate enough vacuum.

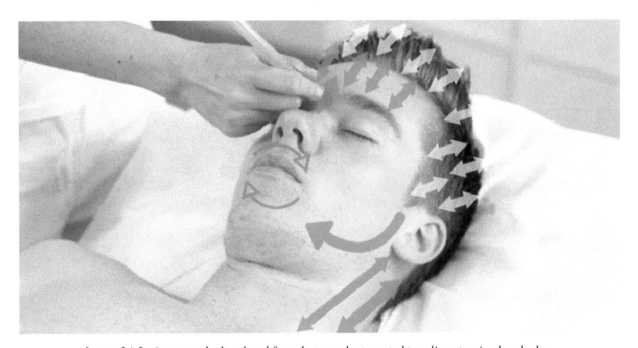

Image 24-2: Areas on the head and face that may be targeted to relieve tension headache.

CERVICAL HEADACHE

Cervical headache is a secondary headache originating from the upper cervical spine, referred from the cervical spine. This is probably due to a misinterpretation by the brain from the afferent nerve signals. Different classifications exist in how to diagnose a cervical headache, but the following is most commonly used:

- Decreased active range of motion of the neck associated with pain in the neck,

- Tender spots in the upper cervical region,

- and unilateral headache.

Usually the lesion or disorder is located from C0 to C3. The headache might also be accompanied with dizziness and nausea.

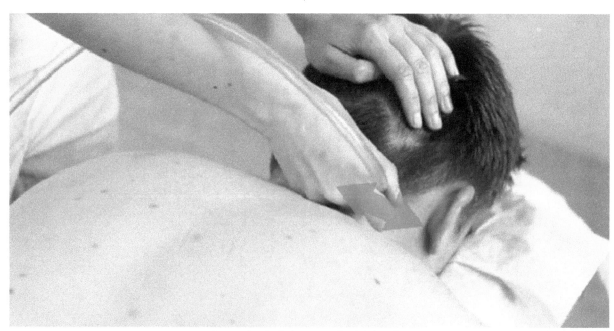

Image 24-3: Release at the C1-level.

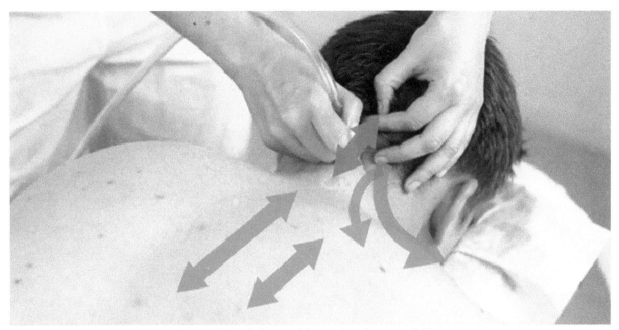

Image 24-4: Release of the occipital area and C2.

Note that scapular muscles like levator scapulae and upper trapezius attach in the upper cervical area, and may contribute to cervicogenic headache. Although only the upper cervical region has the potential to cause a cervicogenic headache, it is advised to treat the entire cervical spine and upper thoracic region, due to the co-contraction and closely related activation patterns of these muscles.

DIZZINESS RELATED TO CERVICAL SPINE

Dizziness, also called vertigo, which is vast subject, is a common problem for many people and may be related to the cervical spine. However, the most common cause of dizziness is Orthostatic Hypotension, where a decrease in blood-pressure causes short-term (usually a few seconds) dizziness. This commonly occurs when standing up quickly.

The source of a patient's dizziness should be verified by a medical doctor before starting any treatment of the patient.

Dizziness often originates from the cervical spine at level C0-3 and general tension around the neck.

Treating the following neck muscles may help the patient. Pay special attention from approximately C5 and proximally:

- Upper trapezius

- Erector spinae

- Levator scapula

- Scalenes/sternocleidomastoideus

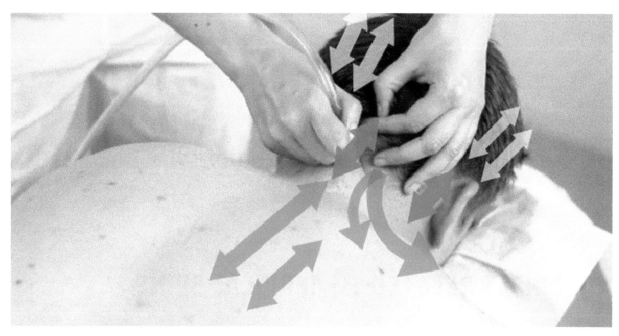

Image 24-5: Figure showing important areas to treat when trying to relieve symptoms of dizziness. Treat the whole back of the neck, specially from C0 to C3. Also, include the attachment of levator scapula and the trapezius.

[25] TREATING THE JAW

Jaw tension is often related to teeth grinding during sleep or while awake. It is also often related to stress. Clicking in the temporomandibular joint may indicate issues with the discoid structure. They may need a dentist to make a night guard for grinding. The most common muscles affecting the jaw are:

- Sternocleidomastoid

- Scalene

- Masseter

- Temporalis

- Pectoralis minor / major

Prolonged jaw pain may cause neck pain.

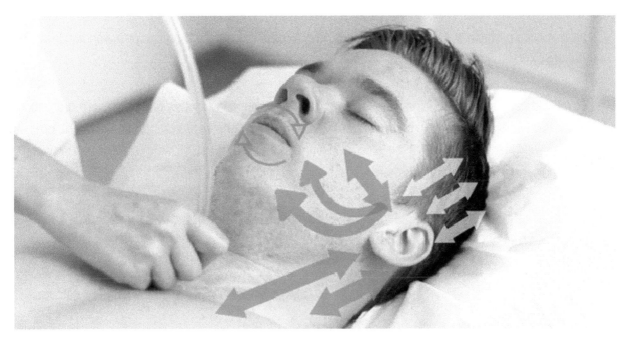

Image 25-1: Important treatment areas for releasing tension around the jaw.

[26] TREATING THE THORACIC SPINE

The thoracic spine is comprised of twelve vertebras, 24 ribs, and the sternum. It connects the lower limb with the upper limb, and has numerous muscles attached to it.

A well-functioning thoracic spine is thereby important, as restricted movement can result in compensatory movements of the cervical and lumbar spine, resulting in injuries in these regions. In sports, sufficient rotation is vital for a pitcher, as the athlete is often forced to compensate with further shoulder motion.

The sympathetic nervous system exits the thoracic spine, which supplies signals to many important organs. Some believe that lesions in the thoracic spine may change the signals that regulates organs, and that this in turn can result in sub-optimal function of various organs.

You may need to treat the thoracic secondary to increase function in the lumbar spine and cervical, as these regions co-relate.

If a patient has a problem with one of the ribs, it is often helpful to treat the thoracic corresponding level, in addition to releasing intercostal muscles.

Try to differentiate between pain from the sterno-costal, intercostal musculature and costo-vertebral joint. Often the patient will describe pain on the site of the actual injury. Otherwise, compression of the rib or vertebra usually result in pain where the injury is located (sternally or dorsally). Pain on palpation between the ribs, indicate pain from the intercostal muscle.

Aerobic exercise is important for the thoracic spine, due to the expansion of the thoracic cage. Self-mobilization, especially including rotation is also helpful.

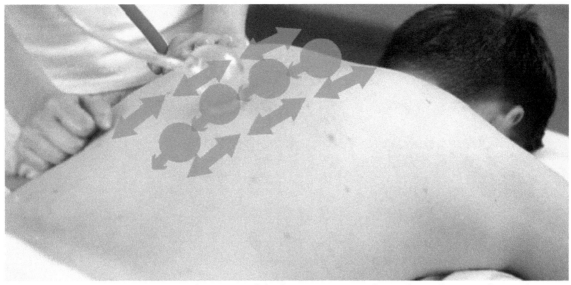

Image 26-1: Demonstrates static techniques with high intensity on each vertebra. Alternatively, try dynamic technique with lateral to medial or longitudinal movements of the cup. Areas with pain, high tension, or increased bruising should be focused.

MUSCLES TO RELEASE THE THORACIC

- Interspinal

- Erector spina and paraspinal

- Intercostal (compresses the ribs together..harder to breath)

- Serratus

- Latissimus (compresses the ribs)

- Rhomboid

- Chest muscles

- Abdominal muscles (makes it harder to extend thoracic)

It may be beneficial to combine treatment with stretching, breathing, and aerobic exercises.

[27] TREATING THE LUMBAR SPINE/PELVIS

Chronic lower back pain is now considered in a bio-psycho-social aspect. But here we will focus on how to help the patient via the muscular-system. Keep in mind that in chronic cases, a multi-disciplinary approach may be needed.

Often the primary driver of pain is the lumbar disc and/or facet joints. These cannot be influenced by vacuum therapy, but a secondary increased muscle tone may be addressed. A spontaneous recovery usually occurs with these injuries, so by decreasing muscle tone and pain you can help the patient until the initial injury is healed.

In chronic cases, patients often have too high activation. By addressing the muscles primarily responsible, a significant pain decrease may be achieved.

Try to asses movement, function and muscles to discover which muscles may contribute to the impairment.

MUSCLES THAT COMMONLY GIVES BACK PAIN

- Psoas

- Iliacus

- Quadratus lumborum

- Latissimus dorsi

- Gluteal

- Diafragma

- Abdominal muscles (may increase the compressional force applied on the spine)

Work towards the thoracic area to relieve secondary tension

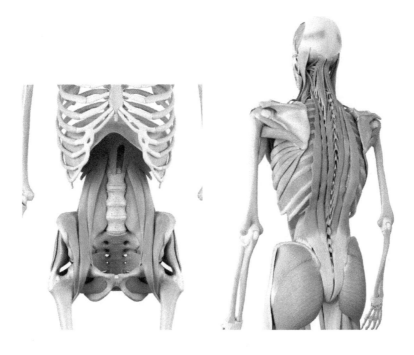

Image 27-1: Important muscles for the lower back

Other recommendations:

- Also work over the vertebra.

- Work over the ligaments around sacrum, especially the long dorsal sacro-iliac ligament.

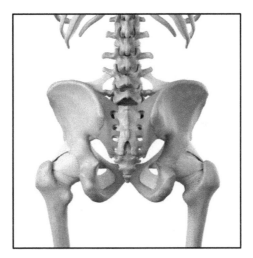

Image 27-2: The ligaments around sacrum and the lumbar vertebras.

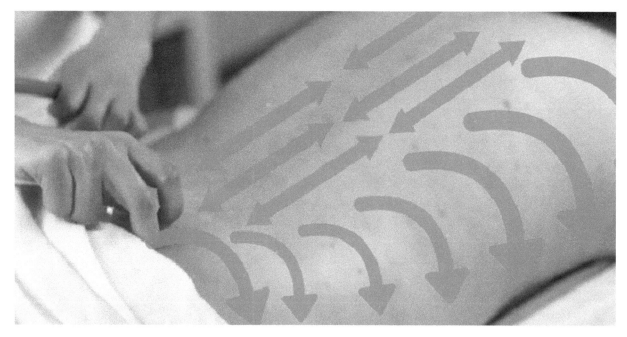

Image 27-3: Treatment areas for relieving the lumbar spine. Start centrally around the lumbar spine. Consider release of the thoracic spine as tension here can result in secondary tension in the lumbar area. Work on the quadratus lumborum, and include the ribcage. Don't forget the ligaments around the sacrum, the gluteal muscles, piriformis and the latissimus dorsi.

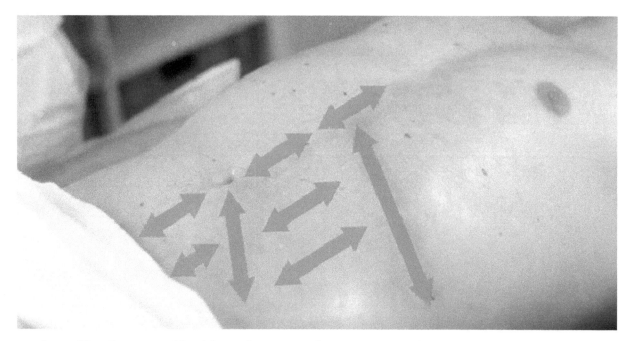

Image 27-4: Treatment of the abdominal area may relieve tension in the lumbar spine. Work on the psoas (indirectly), the diaphragm, rectus abdominis, transversus abdominis and internal/external oblique muscles. Increased tension in the abdominal area may increase tension in the lumbar spine. Prolonged over-activity of muscles surrounding the lumbar spine may decrease flexibility, and result in compressional forces on the lumbar disc and facet-joints.

[28] IMPROVING POSTURE WITH THE TUXEN METHOD

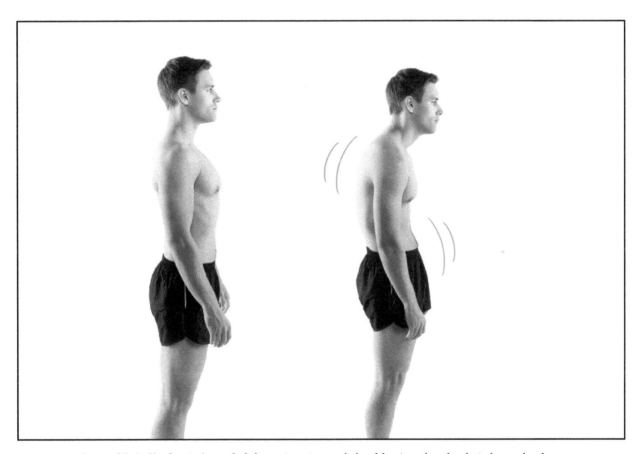

Image 28-1: Kyphosis (rounded thoracic spine and shoulders) and an lordotic lower back.

MUSCLES THAT AFFECT POSTURE

- Latissimus dorsi (compressing the thoracic into curved position)

- Intercostal muscles (may decrease the available expansive movement between the ribs.)

- Diafragma (Increased tone in the diaphragm may result in a sub-optimal breathing pattern.)

- Pectoralis minor and major (tilting the scapula anterior)

- Rhomboid (Often needs to be released to allow optimal scapular movement.)

- Rectus abdominis

- Hamstring (Over-activity of the hamstring may tilt the pelvis into counternutation and cause hyperlordosis in the lumbar spine, and kyphosis in the thoracic spine.)

- Gastrocnemius (often tight due to tight hamstring)

If a female patient over 40 years old displays a significant thoracic kyphosis, be aware of early osteoporosis. Ask the patient to consult their doctor prior to treatment. Bechterew is also a disease that causes kyphosis in the thoracic spine. Patients with respiratory diseases often have rigid spines due to the increased activity of the intercostal muscles.

After treatment, try to manually correct the patient's posture and teach the patient the new posture. Consider administering stretching exercises, deep breathing exercises, and strength training for the erector spinae and the middle and lower trapezius for a long-lasting result. Aerobic exercises will also self-mobilize the ribs as they expand and compress during inhalation.

IMPROVING THE LORDOTIC LOWER BACK

Muscles to release:

- Psoas (tilting the pelvis into lordosis/nutation)

- Rectus femoris/quadriceps (tilting the pelvis into lordosis)

- Erector spinae (overextending the lower back

- Latissimus dorsi (general compressing force)

Correct patient's posture manually after releasing the muscles and teach the patient how to stand correctly. Consider stretching exercises for the most compromised muscles. Also, consider strengthening exercises to enhance the effect. Usually it is beneficial to strengthen antagonists to the muscles that you have released. For example, release psoas, and strengthen the hamstring.

BEAUTY & HYGENE

[29] CELLULITE

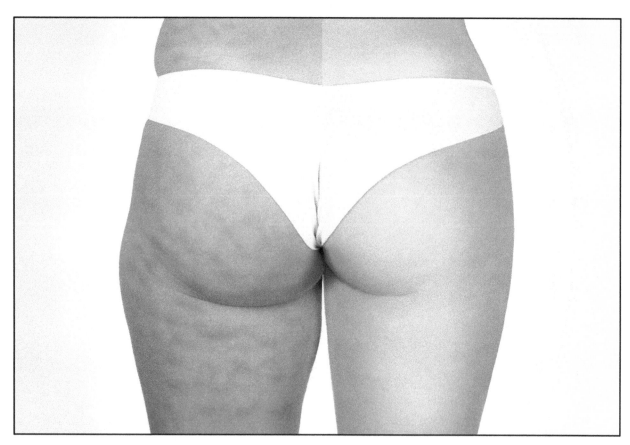

Image 29-1: A comparison of cellulite (left side) versus no cellulite (the right side).

WHAT IS CELLULITE?

Cellulite is very common in women, in fact, almost all women have some degree of cellulite, even skinny women. Cellulite is nothing more than fat cells pushing against the connective tissue giving it an uneven, dimpled, and lumpy appearance. Cellulite forms easiest in areas with poor circulation, so without activity and exercise it is very hard to eradicate.

Women get more cellulite than men because they generally have more fat and estrogen, but the main reason is that the bands connecting skin and muscle are different in men than they are in women. Men have thicker bands, more of them, and they form a crisscross pattern as opposed to the vertical pattern on women's bodies. This keeps the fat in place so it doesn't bulge the same way it does on women.

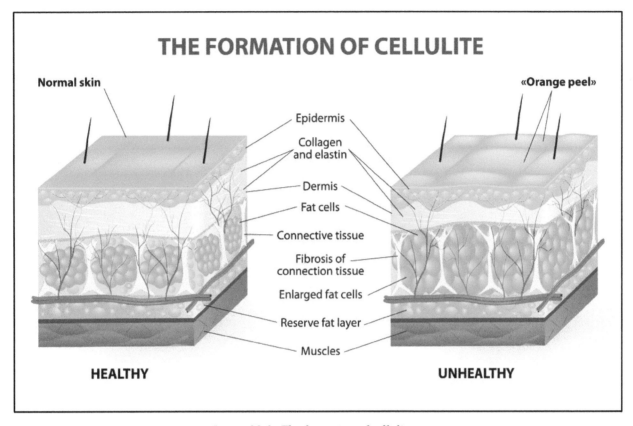

Image 29-2: The formation of cellulite

The best way to get rid of cellulite is to be regularly physically active and to eat healthy, whole foods with a minimum of processed and artificial foods as they create a lot of waste and can make the body retain water, fording the body to store these toxins in the fat cells.

An effective way to treat cellulite is to use the Tuxen Method vacuum therapy to increase circulation, improve the lymph system, and help the fat cells get rid of waste products. Exercise is also recommended, along with weight loss if the person is overweight.

COMMON SIDE EFFECTS

The Tuxen Method cellulite treatment can help assist weight loss. The treatment helps the body to get rid of toxins and improve lymph drainage and often a person carries a lot of stored up fluid in their tissue, not just fat. As a patient rids his or herself of the released toxins, they can often feel tired through the day after treatment, feel that they have to urinate more often, and find that the urine smells differently.

Acupuncture meridians that stimulate the metabolism are also stimulated during treatment. Very often this has a positive effect on energy and weight loss (if needed). Skinny people can also benefit in terms of more even connective tissue, increased energy, and a feeling of lighter legs.

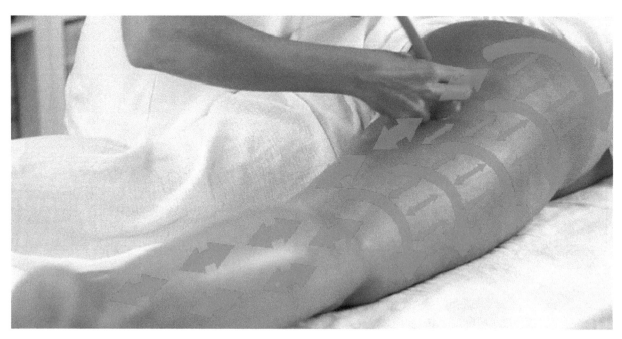

Image 29-3: Cellulite treatment. Use as much vacuum pressure as the client can handle and move up and down and sideways to stimulate the tissue in as many directions as possible. Work on front and back of the body. This approach can be used anywhere there is cellulite, like the stomach and arms in addition to the legs.

[30] STRETCH MARKS

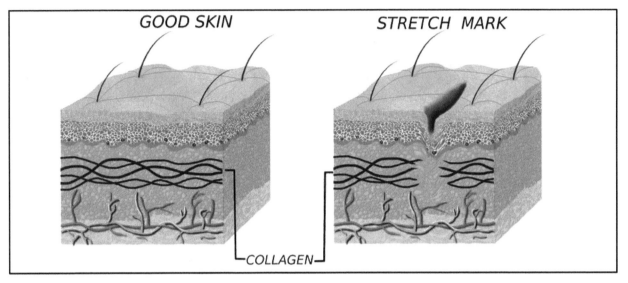

Image 30-1: Skin where the collagen fibers are broken and a stretch mark is created. Collagen fibers often get broken when they are forced to stretch quicker and beyond their limits of elasticity. The quality of collagen is also influenced by diet and lifestyle.

WHAT ARE STRETCH MARKS?

Stretch marks are long, narrow streaks, stripes or lines that develop on the skin and which differ in hue from the surrounding skin. They are the result of a sudden stretching of the skin and are extremely common. Anyone can develop stretch marks, although they tend to affect more women than men. Stretch marks are not medically dangerous, but they can cause an aesthetic concern. For some people, stretch marks are a significant cosmetic concern.

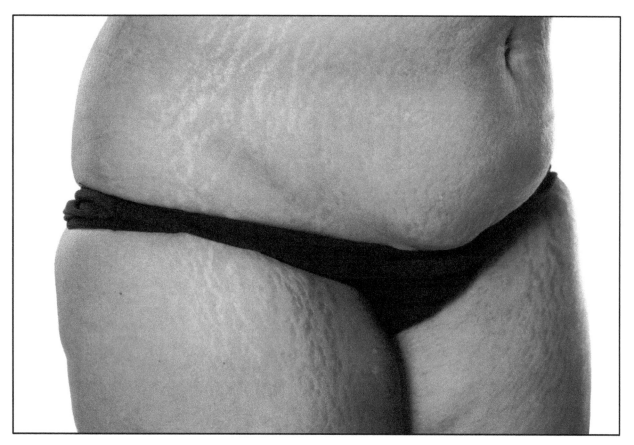

Image 30-2: Woman with stretch marks on thighs and stomach.

The Tuxen Method stimulates the connective tissue for collagen renewal and this may reduce the appearance of stretch marks. With treatment, the skin inside the stretch marks may become very bruised and the stretch marks might seem highlighted, but after a few days the healing will make the skin firm up and the stretch marks will appeared to have reduced.

When treating stretch marks with the Tuxen Method use a *small* cup and as *high pressure* on the vacuum as the person can handle. Work with quick and short strokes, and try to produce bruising in as much of the surface skin as possible. This will create a strong regeneration impulse of the upper layers of the skin and help the collagen fiber material to rebuild and renew itself.

This process stimulates collagen renewal, increases skin elasticity, and firms it up. It also increases nutrition to the skin through increased blood circulation.

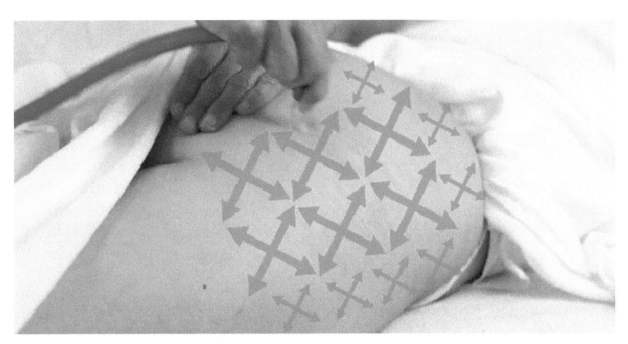

Image 30-3: The Tuxen Method in improving the appearance of stretch marks. The small cup is used with maximum pressure on the vacuum machine and moved with short strokes in every direction to produce bruising in as much of the surface skin as possible to force a strong regeneration process in the skin layers after treatment.

[31] ECZEMA

Optimization of lymph flow and circulation can help improve eczema and other skin conditions after regular treatments. This is a very common "side effect" that many of our patients have discovered if they have come to our clinic for other problems such as neck and shoulder pain, and their skin condition has improved in addition to having relief of the neck and shoulder, for example.

Tuxen Method is different from other lymph stimulation therapies because it increases and optimizes the capillaries so that the lymph system is greatly improved, even long after treatment. The Tuxen Method does not just move lymph, it helps the underlying cause of reduced lymph flow.

Many people with eczema have skin with poor circulation and poor lymph flow. Use a small cup and as high pressure on the vacuum as the person can handle and try to produce bruising in as much of the surface skin as possible. This will create a strong regeneration impulse of the upper skin layers, reduce inflammation, improve circulation, and permanently improve the lymph flow so that the skin has a better ability to stay healthy.

You might also advise the patient to talk to a nutritionist to make sure their diet and nutrition is optimized. Any autoimmune condition worsens with stress, so if the patient is stressed you might advise them to seek help managing their stress levels.

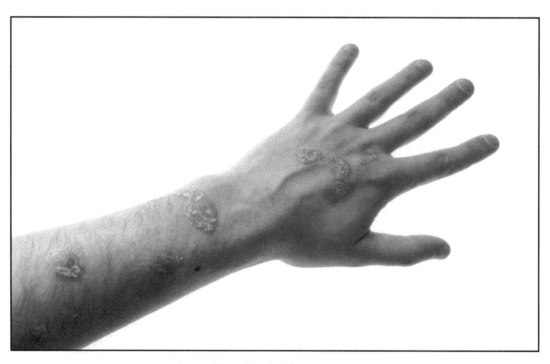

Image 29-x: Hand with eczema spots.

[32] FACE LIFT

The Tuxen Method can help give a "facelift" because of the effect from the breakdown of the tissue which forces it to renew itself with improved circulation and collagen structures. This is the same stimuli that much more expensive treatments attempt, such as CO2 laser treatments.

When you have given a treatment with the Tuxen Method on the face and neck there will be some "down time" where the patient may look worse and may want to stay indoors 3-4 days, or may want to cover the bruises with makeup. This is unavoidable with any treatment that gives a similar strong effect and the downtime from the Tuxen Method is much less than the downtime from C02 lasers, for example.

You can also obtain a benefit of "shredding" the top layers of the skin if you recommend the patient does a face scrub with sugar and lemon every 2-3 days over a few weeks between the treatments. Just add lemon juice to a cotton ball, add sugar, then rub it over the face and neck or any area that you want to peel. This will create a new glow and dim pigmentation spots in addition to firming up the area treated.

Image 32-1: Suggested directions for facelift. Follow suggested direction but be aware that the main effect comes from the breakdown of the tissue (which forces it to renew itself and improve circulation and collagen structures). This effect comes independent of direction.

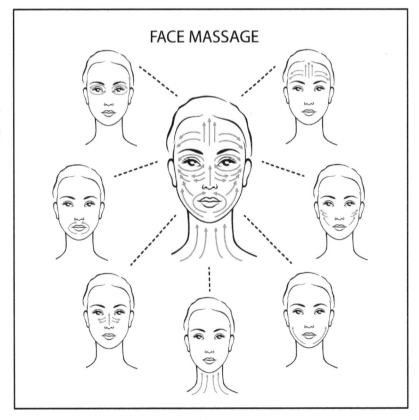

FACE MASSAGE

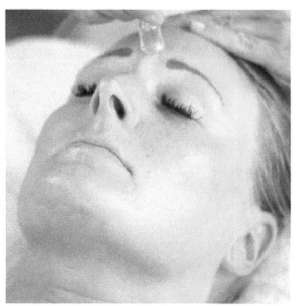 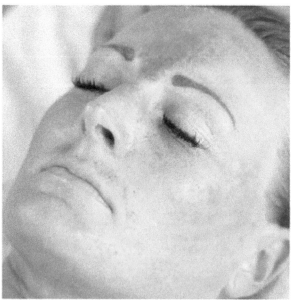

Image 32-2: Patient before and right after a facelift treatment. The patient has bruised in the areas where there was most tension. The bruised areas are typically the areas that will improve the most after treatment, but the whole face will benefit and get firmer and the appearance of fine lines and wrinkles may improve to a very visible degree.

[33] BLACKHEADS

Blackheads are small bumps that appear on the skin due to clogged hair follicles. These bumps are called "blackheads" because the surface looks dark or black. Blackheads are a mild type of acne.

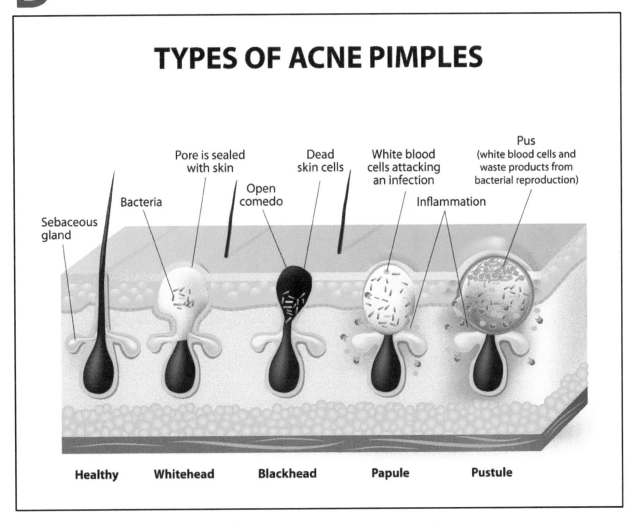

Image 33-1: Figure of blackhead and other types of acne.

Tuxen Method on blackheads is simply using the power of a strong vacuum machine to suck the black head straight out. The method is highly effective and comfortable for the patient. Before you try to suck the blackhead out from the skin it is very effective to do a light peeling first to get rid of the dead skin that might work as a "lid" keeping the blackhead sealed. As discussed, the most effective scrub is a combination of sugar and lemon. Just add lemon juice to a cotton ball and then add sugar and rub it over the area that you want to peel. After this, simply apply oil and use a small vacuum cup with as high pressure as possible on your machine. Start to move the cup in circular movements around the blackhead. In just a few seconds the blackhead will pop.

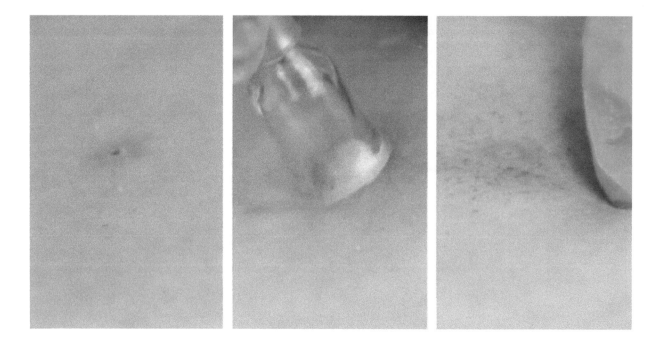

Image 33-2: First figure is of blackhead after it has been scrubbed with lemon and sugar. Second figure is showing the vacuum cup moving in circles over the blackhead and the last figure shows that the blackhead has been sucked out and there is just a empty hole.

FURTHER STUDY

[34] ACUPUNCTURE MERIDIANS AND REFLEXOLOGY POINTS

WHAT ARE ACUPUNCTURE MERIDIANS AND REFLEXOLOGY POINTS?

Meridians are a network of channels that transport an organ's electrical energy. Acupuncture points are areas where the electrical energy is best accessible for stimulation. Most acupuncture points are placed along meridians, but they can also manifest other places outside the meridian, such as the foot, hand, and ear reflexology points. We have 12 meridians—10 represent organs, 2 represent functions (circulation and hormonal system).

STIMULATING MERIDIANS WITH THE TUXEN METHOD

Organs that are "out of balance" manifest as tension on the skin surface of the meridian. The function of an organ can be influenced by the stimulation of the acupuncture points on the meridian. When you balance the tension in the meridian, the organ also seems to get back into balance.

The tension on the outside (skin) of the body is somehow connected to the tension on the inside of the body. We get a feeling of what is happening on the inside by analyzing the outside surface, and assessing meridian tension is a very old and traditional way of doing this.

A very powerful stimulation of a meridian is achieved by using Tuxen Method on the meridian or directly on the acupuncture point. Simply follow the meridian with a small vacuum cup with high pressure, and if there is a lot of tension you want to release this tension by moving the vacuum cup up and down and in every direction until the tension is released or the area is nice and red. If there is a lot of difference between the meridian area on the right versus the left side if the body (meridians normally run parallel on both the left and right sides of the body), you want to spend a longer time on the most painful side.

MERIDIAN POINTS, THEIR SYMPTOMS AND CHARACTERISTICS

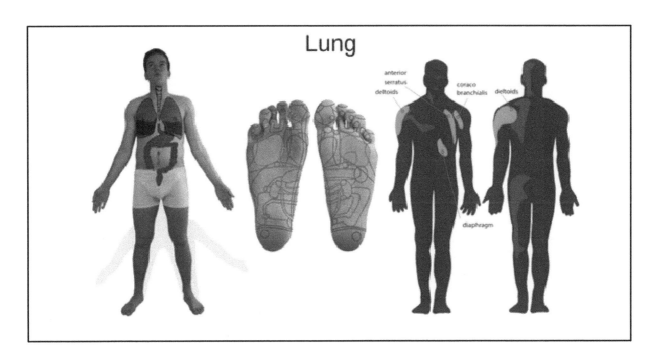

Image 34-1: Lung meridian with foot reflexology point and associated muscles.

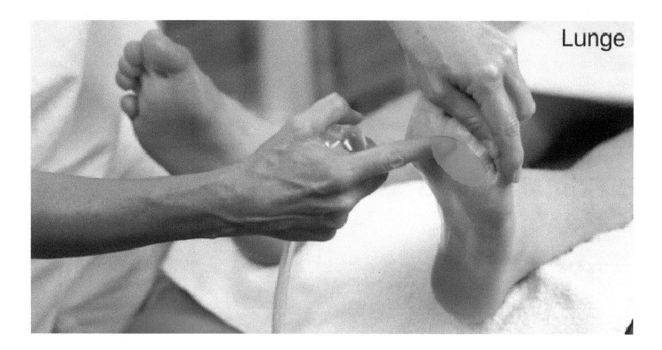

Image 34-2: Lung area on foot. Area is located on both the right and left foot.

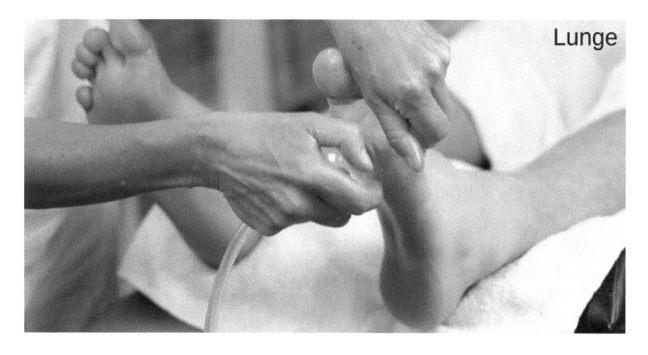

Image 34-3: How to treat the Lunge foot reflexology point with the Tuxen Method.

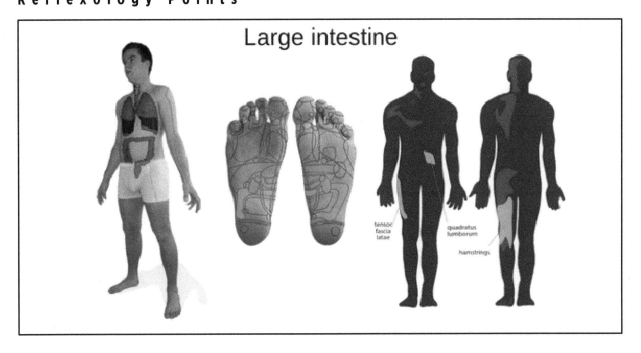

Image 34-4: Large intestine meridian with foot reflexology point and associated muscles.

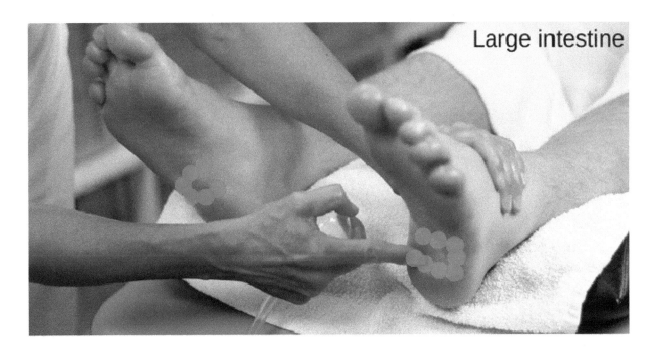

Image 34-5: Large intestine area on foot. Area is located on both the right and left foot.

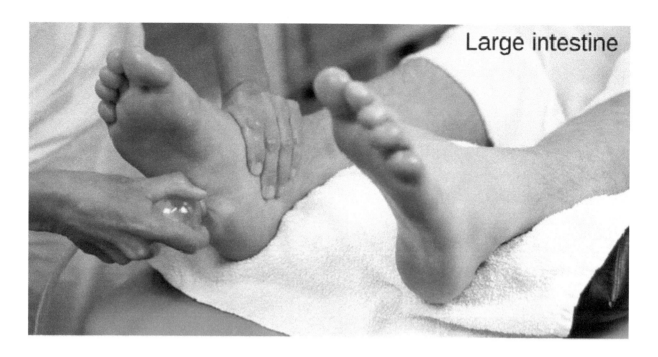

Image 34-6: Treatment with the Tuxen Method.

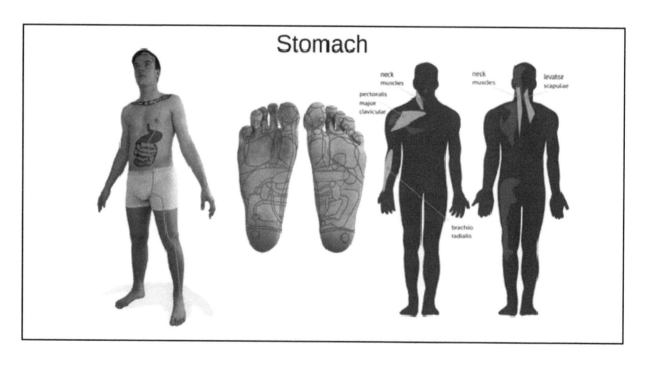

Image 34-7: Stomach meridian with foot reflexology point and associated muscles.

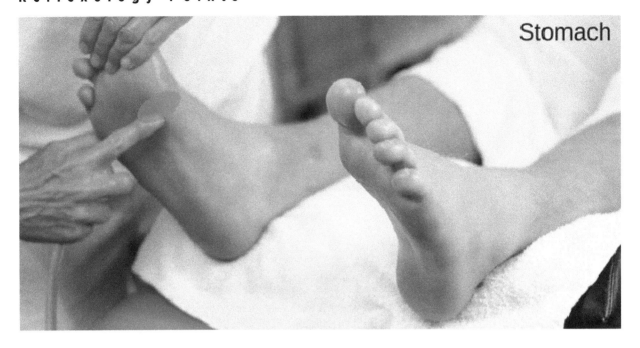

Image 34-8: Stomach area on foot. Area is located on both the right and left foot.

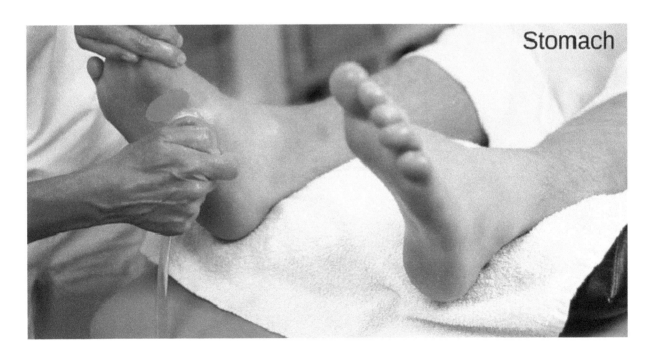

Image 34-9: Treatment with the Tuxen Method.

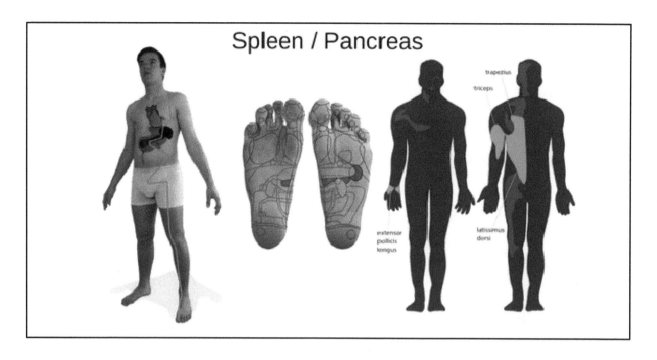

Image 34-10: Spleen/Pancreas meridian with foot reflexology point and associated muscles.

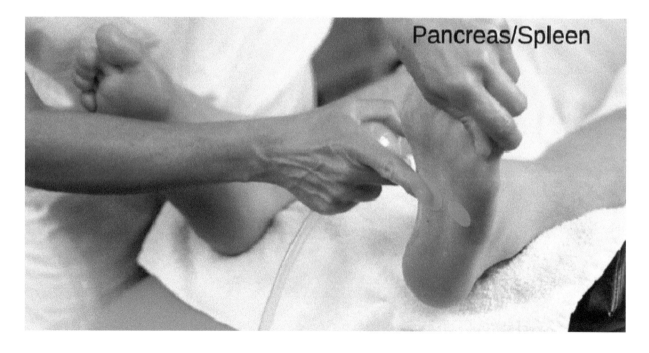

Image 34-11: Pancreas/spleen area on foot. Area is located on mainly on the left foot since the pancreas and spleen mainly lies on the left side of the body.

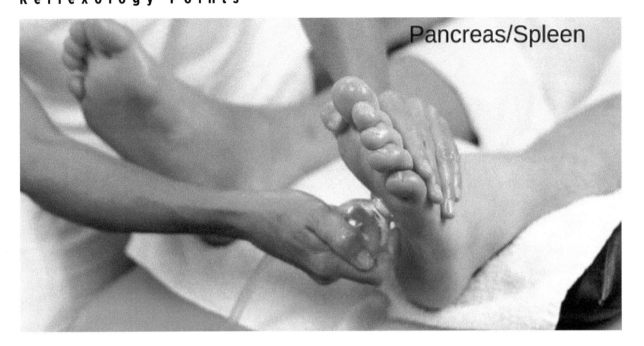

Image 34-12: Treatment with the Tuxen Method.

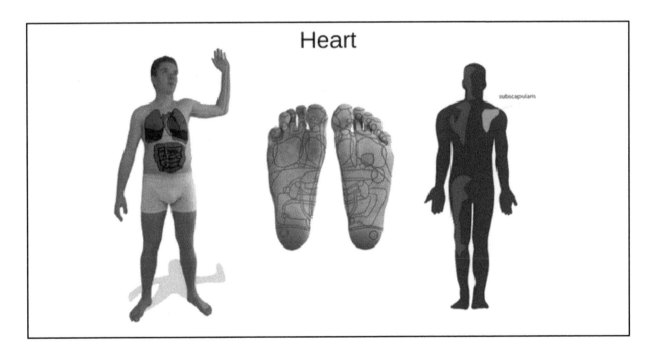

*Image 34-13: **Heart meridian** with foot reflexology point and associated muscles.*

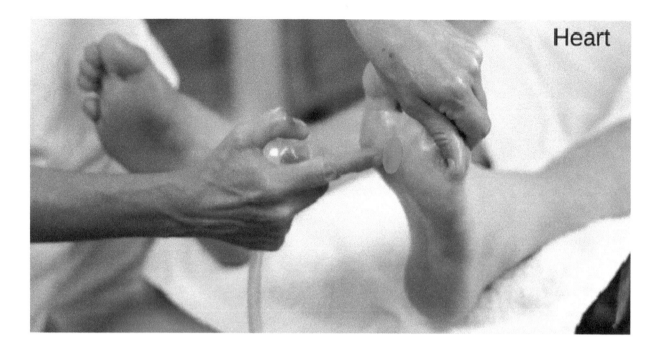

Image 34-14: The Heart area on foot. Area is located on the left foot.

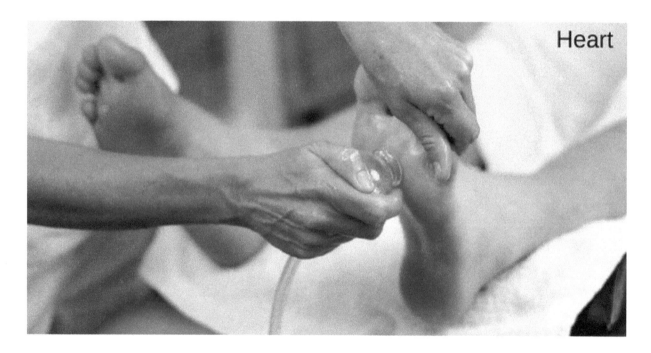

Image 34-15: Treatment with the Tuxen Method.

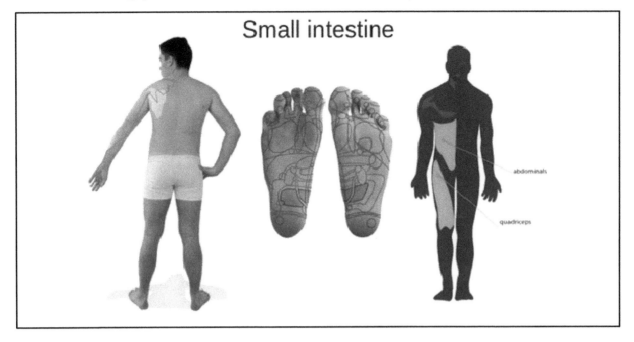

Image 34-16: Small intestine meridian with foot reflexology point and associated muscles.

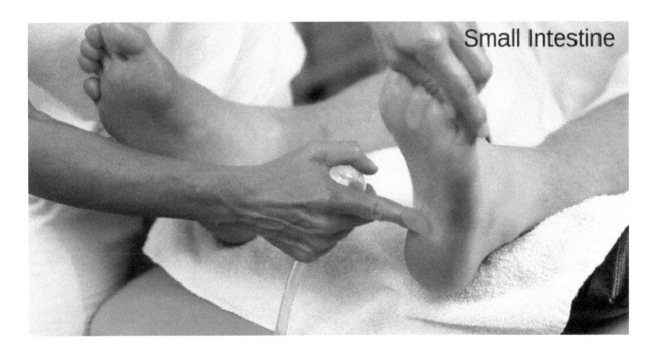

Image 34-17: Tthe Small intestine area on foot. Area is located on both the right and left foot.

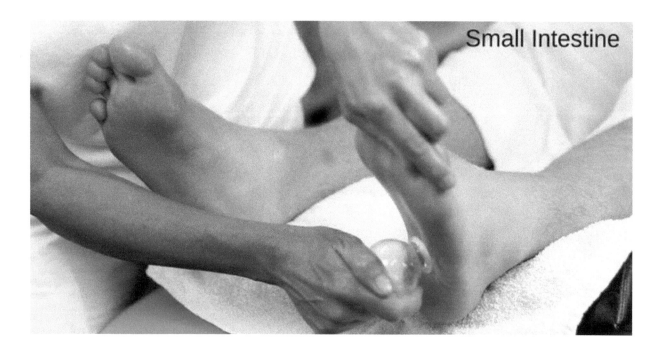

Image 34-18: Treatment with the Tuxen Method.

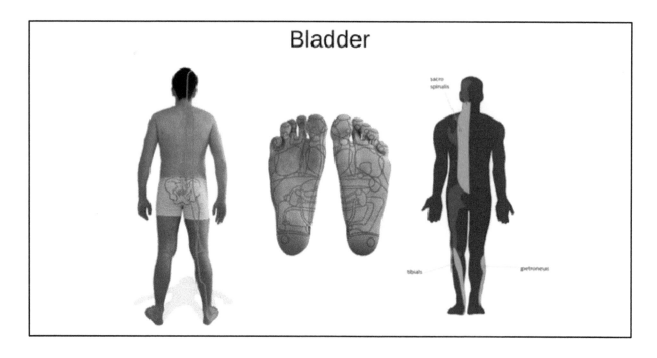

Image 34-19: Bladder meridian with foot reflexology point and associated muscles.

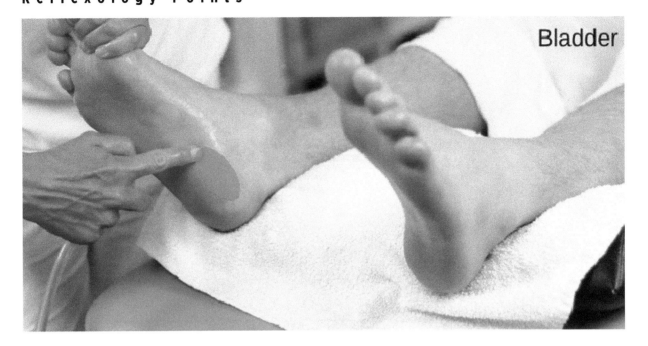

Image 34-20: The Bladder area on foot. Area is located on both the right and left foot.

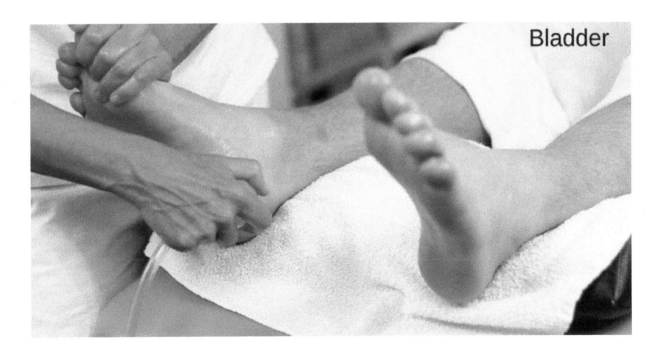

Image 34-21: Treatment with the Tuxen Method.

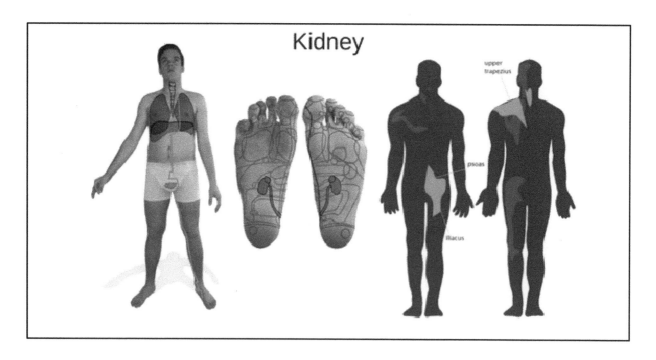

Image 34-22: Kidney meridian with foot reflexology point and associated muscles.

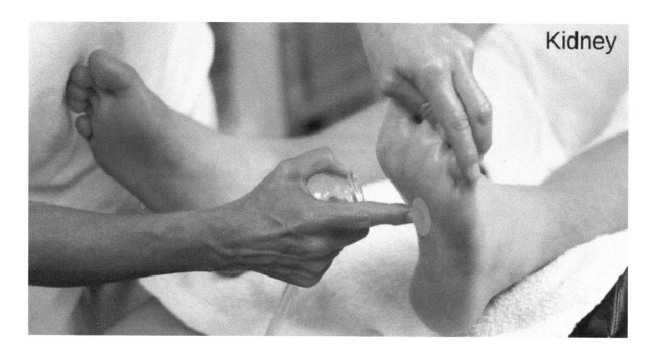

Image 34-23: The kidney area on foot. Area is located on both the right and left foot.

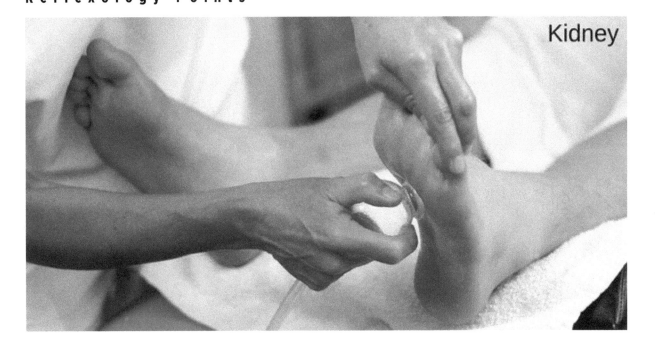

Image 34-24: Treatment with the Tuxen Method.

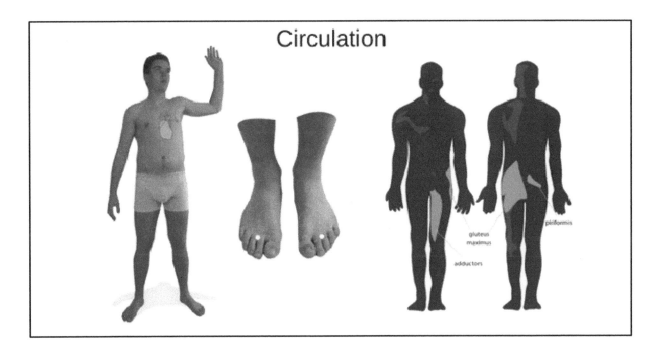

Image 34-25: Circulation meridian with foot reflexology point and associated muscles.

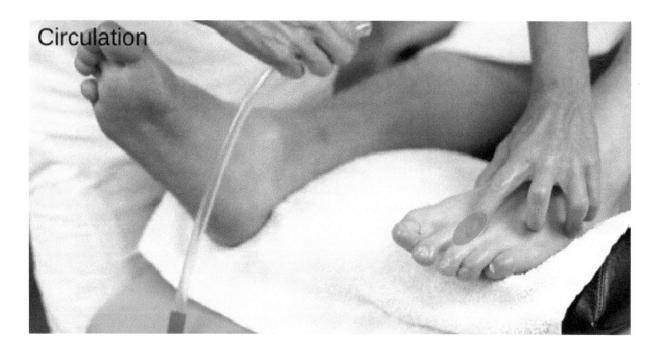

Image 34-26: The circulation area on the foot. The area is located on both the right and left foot.

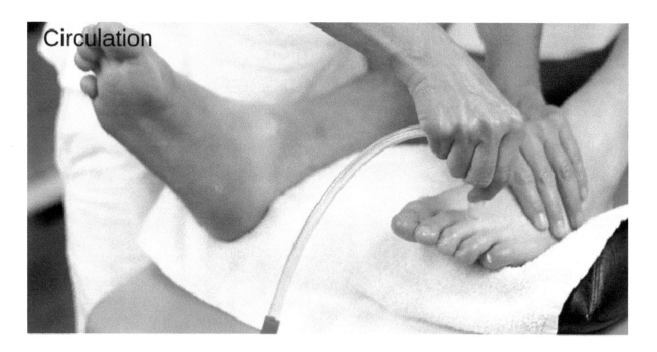

Image 34-27: Treatment with the Tuxen Method.

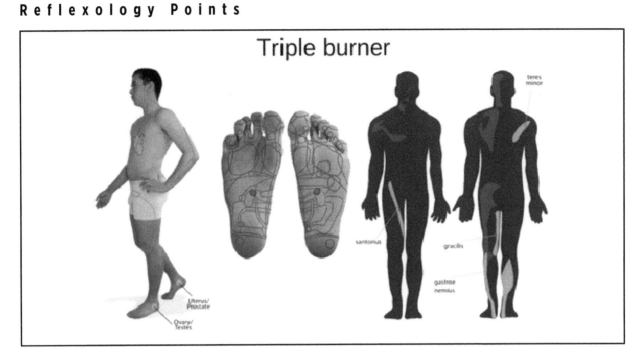

Image 34-28: Triple burner meridian with foot reflexology point and associated muscles.

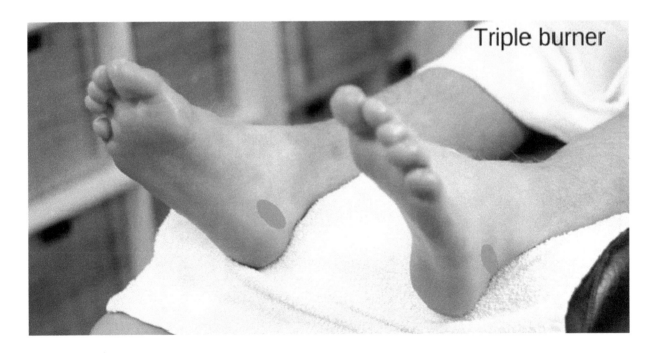

Image 34-29: The ovaries/prostate area on foot. Area is located on both the right and left foot.

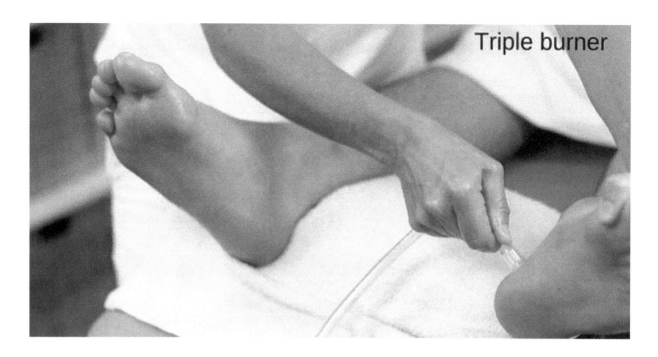

Image 34-30: Treatment with the Tuxen Method.

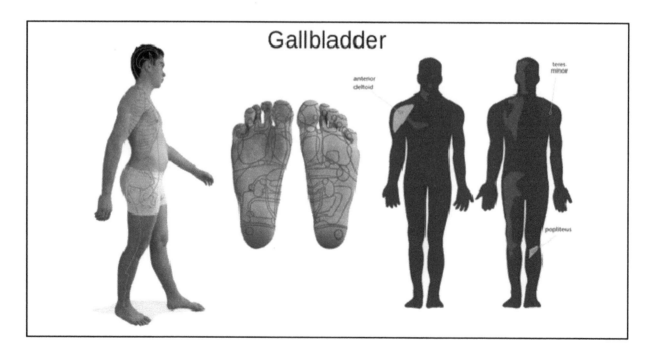

Image 34-31: Gallbladder meridian with foot reflexology point and associated muscles.

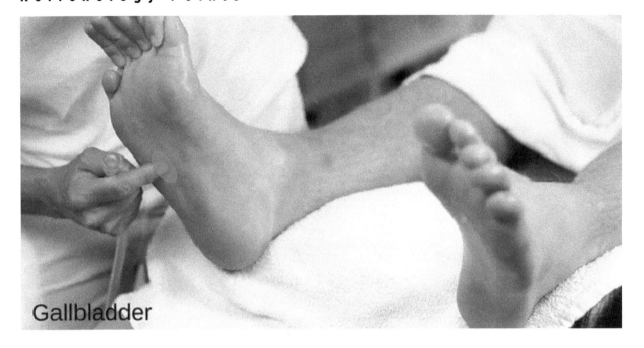

Image 34-32: The Gallbladder area on foot. Area is located only on the right foot.

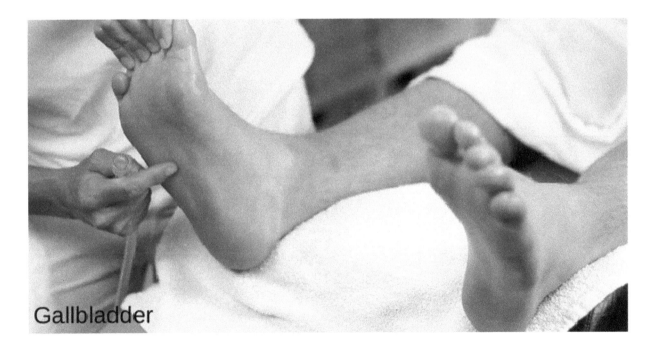

Image 34-33: Treatment with the Tuxen Method.

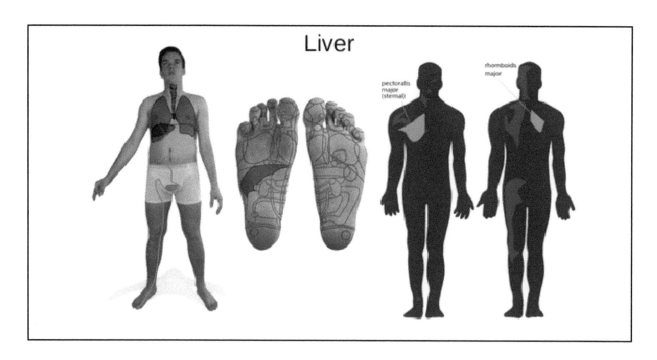

Image 34-34: Liver meridian with foot reflexology point and associated muscles.

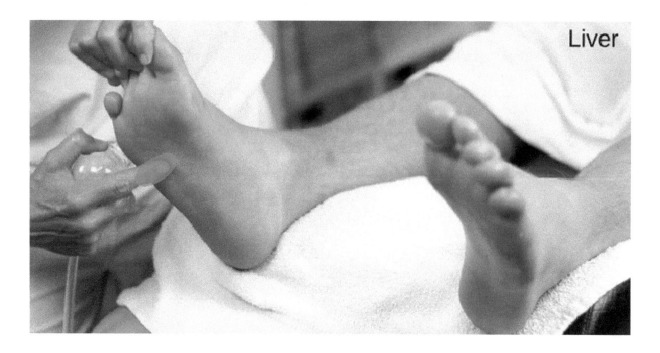

Image 34-35: The Liver area on foot. Area is located only on the right foot.

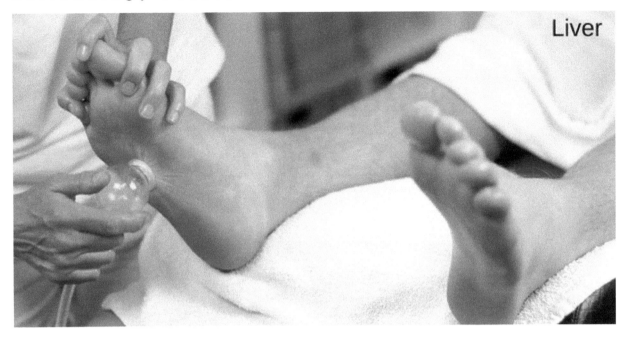

Image 34-36: Treatment with the Tuxen Method.

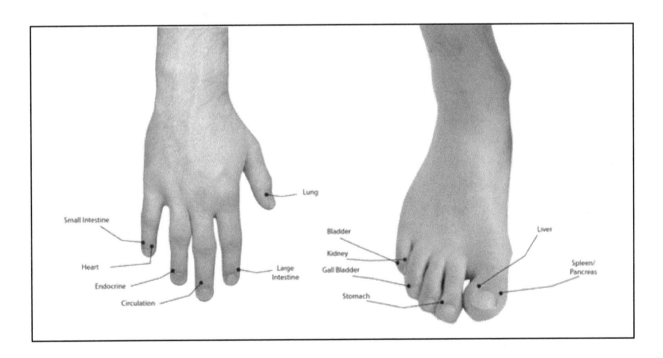

Image 34-37: Meridian endings

LEARN MORE!

For a FREE downloadable wall poster of all figures please visit

www.tuxenmethod.com/products

IMPORTANT!

Patients with life-threatening diseases and serious medical problems should always consult their doctor before receiving vacuum therapy. Avoid any area that has cancer or is infected. Avoid the abdominal area during pregnancy and be more gentle and careful when applying vacuum therapy to a pregnant woman. If any area hurts excessively, use a light pressure/vacuum instead. Use a lighter pressure in the lymph area such as the throat, groin, below the ears, and the outer breast near the armpits. Do not vacuum treat directly on a serious burn or radiation area until it has healed. Ulcerous conditions and infections should receive medical care. Do not work directly on a recently formed scar or tumor. Never do vacuum therapy under the influence of alcohol or drugs.

PERSONAL RESPONSIBILITY AND ASSUMPTION OF RISK

As a Licensee, you agree that you are using your own judgment in using our Programs, Products, Services and Program Materials and you agree that you are doing so at your own risk. Our Programs, Products, Services and Program Materials are for informational and educational purposes only. You agree and understand that you assume all risks and no results are guaranteed in any way related to our Programs, Products, Services and Program Materials. Our Programs, Products, Services and Program Materials are merely to provide you with education and tools to help you make your own decisions. You are solely responsible for your actions, decisions and results based on the use, misuse or non-use of our Programs, Products,

Services and Program Materials, and if you are a practitioner yourself, you are solely responsible for exercising your own judgment in applying what you have learned from our Programs, Products, Services and Program Materials, and you alone are solely responsible for your clients/patients actions and results.

We take every precaution to protect our Programs, Products, Services and Program Materials. However, due to the nature of the Internet, we cannot completely ensure or warrant the security of the Programs, Products, Services and Program Materials or the contributions or information transmitted to us on or through our Website or our Programs, Products, Services and Program Materials. Submitting contributions or information on our through our Programs, Products, Services and Program Materials is done entirely at your own risk. We make no assurances about our ability to prevent any such loss or damage to you or to any other person, company or entity arising out of use of our Programs, Products, Services and Program Materials and you agree that you are assuming such risks.

DISCLAIMERS

Our Programs, Products, Services, and Program Materials are for informational and educational purposes only. To the fullest extent permitted by law, we expressly exclude any liability for any direct, indirect or consequential loss or damage incurred by you, your clients/patients, or others in connection with our Programs, Products, Services, and Program Materials, including without limitation any liability for any accidents, delays, injuries, harm, loss, damage, death, lost profits, personal or business interruptions, misapplication of information, physical or mental disease, condition or issue, physical, mental, emotional, or spiritual injury or harm, loss of income or revenue, loss of business, loss of profits or contracts, anticipated savings, loss of data, loss of goodwill, wasted time and for any other loss or damage of any kind, however and whether caused by negligence, breach of contract, or otherwise, even if foreseeable. You specifically acknowledge and agree that we are not liable for any defamatory, offensive or illegal conduct of any other Program, Product, Service or Program Materials participant or user, including you.

Medical Disclaimer. Our Programs, Products, Services, and Program Materials are not to be perceived as or relied upon in any way as medical advice or mental health advice. The information provided through our Programs, Products, Services, and Program Materials is not intended to be a substitute for professional medical advice, diagnosis or treatment that can be provided by your own physician, nurse practitioner, physician assistant, therapist, counselor, mental health practitioner, licensed dietitian or nutritionist, member of the clergy, or any other licensed or registered healthcare professional. We are not providing health care, medical or nutrition therapy services or attempting to diagnose, treat, prevent or cure in any manner whatsoever any physical ailment, or any mental or emotional issue, disease or condition of yours, or if you are a practitioner yourself, in any of your clients or patients. We are not giving medical, psychological, or religious advice whatsoever through our Programs, Products, Services, and Program Materials. You and your clients/patients should always seek the advice of your own Medical Provider and/or Mental Health Provider regarding any questions or concerns you have about your or their specific health or any medications, herbs or supplements you or they are currently taking and before implementing any recommendations or suggestions from our Programs, Products, Services, and Program Materials. You and your clients/patients should not disregard medical advice or delay seeking medical

advice because of information you have read or received in our Programs, Products, Services, and Program Materials. You and your clients/patients should not start or stop taking any medications without speaking to your and their, respectively, own Medical Provider or Mental Health Provider. If you or your clients/patients have or suspect that you have a medical or mental health problem, contact your own Medical Provider or Mental Health Provider promptly.

Legal and Financial Disclaimer. Our Programs, Products, Services, and Program Materials are not to be perceived or relied upon in any way as business, financial or legal advice. The information provided through our Programs, Products, Services, and Program Materials is not intended to be a substitute for professional advice that can be provided by your own accountant, lawyer, or financial advisor. We are not giving financial or legal advice in any way. Although care has been taken in preparing the information provided through our Programs, Products, Services, and Program Materials, we cannot be held responsible for any errors or omissions, and we accept no liability whatsoever for any loss or damage you or your clients/patients may incur. You and your clients/patients should always seek financial and/or legal counsel relating to your specific circumstances as needed for any and all questions and concerns you now have, or may have in the future. You agree that the information provided in or through our Programs, Products, Services, and Program Materials is not legal or financial advice.

Earnings Disclaimer. You acknowledge that we have not and do not make any representations as to the health physical, mental, emotional, spiritual or health benefits, future income, expenses, sales volume or potential profitability or loss of any kind that may be derived as a result of use of our Programs, Products, Services, and Program Materials. We cannot and do not guarantee that you or anyone else, including your clients/patients, will attain a particular result, positive or negative, financial or otherwise, through the use of our

Programs, Products, Services, and Program Materials and you accept and understand that results differ for each individual. We also expressly disclaim responsibility in any way for the choices, actions, results, use, misuse or non-use of the information provided or obtained through the use of our Programs, Products, Services, and Program Materials that is used by you, or that you learn from this Website and share with your clients/patients.

You agree that your results, as well as those of your clients, patients, or anyone else associated with your family or business, are strictly your own responsibility and we are not liable or responsible in any way for your results.

If you have any questions about any term of these Terms of Use, please contact us at support@tuxenmethod.com. Thank you.

EXPANDED CONTENTS